DEPRESSION

Strategies for Managing Anxiety and Depression

(A Vital Guide on How to Deal With Nerves and Coping With Stress)

Norma Rohde

I0146725

Published By Zoe Lawson

Norma Rohde

All Rights Reserved

Depression: Strategies for Managing Anxiety and Depression (A Vital Guide on How to Deal With Nerves and Coping With Stress)

ISBN 978-1-77485-348-1

Legal & Disclaimer

The information contained in this book is not designed to replace or take the place of any form of medicine or professional medical advice. The information in this book has been provided for educational and entertainment purposes only.

The information contained in this book has been compiled from sources deemed reliable, and it is accurate to the best of the Author's knowledge; however, the Author cannot guarantee its accuracy and validity and cannot be held liable for any errors or omissions. Changes are periodically made to this book. You must consult your doctor or get professional medical advice before using any of the suggested remedies, techniques, or information in this book.

TABLE OF CONTENTS

Introduction

In a world that is rife with stress and daily tensions it is evident that individuals will be prone to depression.

According to the findings of a recent study, kids at the age of 6 are beginning to show signs of anxiety as a result of the pressures they have to face throughout their lives. The amount is expected to fall with time.

From kids to professionals working and even busy housewives, everyone is stressed due to one cause or the other , so the requirement for the present is to seek out effective solutions to this issue. If you're one of those who are having difficult times dealing with stress and are unable to fight depression, then you've found the right spot.

This guidebook provides the most effective strategies and steps to aid you in battling depression and help you lead a fulfilling and healthy life.

We will look at the many reasons for depression, and then explore what it means to be and not be depressed.

Chapter 1: An Overview Of Depression

Contrary to what a lot of people think that depression is not just the feeling of sadness. It's more than it seems. It's a medical condition which can significantly affect your life quality. If it is not treated it can become debilitating.

Although it is normal to feel down occasionally, it's not typical to endure long-term sadness. Depression isn't just detrimental to your health, but it may also affect those around you like your friends, family members, and even your coworkers.

Depression can have a devastating effect on both your personal and professional life. It can cause a breakdown in your relationships with friends and family and can even impact your professional career. Depression can cause people to become less productive and disengaged. This leads to many more issues in the future term.

According to the statistics according to statistics, depression is among the most frequent mental health issues worldwide and affects 6.7 percent of the people within The United States. Research has revealed that females are 70 percent more likely to experience depression than men, while non-Hispanic blacks are 40 percent less likely to be affected by depression than whites who are non-Hispanic.

Although depression is more common in older adults, with the median age of at 32, it's additionally found in 3.3 percent of adolescents 13-18 years old. According to the World Health Organization states that major depression is the most frequent form of depression. It accounts for 8.3 percent of all years of life with disability (YLD) in addition to 3.7 percent of the disabled-adjusted lives (DALY).

Depression can worsen when it is suppressed. That is the reason why those who suffer from depression shouldn't try to suppress it. Instead, they should seek help from a professional and get help. Depression is a disease which requires treatment the same way as other major illness. It is not a good idea to think that depression will just disappear by itself.

Depression as experienced by individuals of all ages

Depression can affect any person regardless of gender, age or race. Yet, individuals from different age groups are likely to suffer from depression in different degrees.

Depression in children and Adolescents

Teens and children who suffer from depression tend to carry the illness throughout adulthood. They suffer from the same symptoms as they get older. If they are not treated quickly, they may be diagnosed with other serious illnesses in conjunction with depression.

Children's the inability to attend school and inability to interact with classmates are typical signs of depression. Depression-afflicted children tend to stay away from classes , pretending to be sick or throwing anger issues. They also may be worried about their parents leaving their home or dying. This can make them emotional, anxious and even problematic. They might also feel they are not understood by other people.

However, it isn't always easy to identify the symptoms and signs for depression among children since they often appear like normal behavior of children in this age. Many children experience mood swings and this is an inevitable part of growing up.

However, before they reach the age of adolescence, they generally experience similar depression. As they reach 15 years old However, girls are twice as likely to be suffering from major depression than boys.

As puberty progresses the girls and boys start to confront issues about their

6

sexuality and identities. They also are more likely to be suffering from depression when they begin to make their own choices. As adolescents, depression tends to comes with other health issues such as substance abuse anxieties, eating disorder and a higher risk of suicide.

Depression among women

Certain aspects are known to contribute to depression that women experience. These are factors like hormones, cycles of life as well as psychological and biological aspects. The research suggests that hormones directly affect brain chemistry which regulates moods and emotions of women.

Women are in fact more susceptible to depression following the birth of a child. The type of depression that is known as postpartum depression. It's caused by physical and hormonal aspects of the female body. Many women also get stressed by their new obligations that they face.

Additionally, there are women who suffer from premenstrual syndrome (PMS) or premenstrual dysphoric disorders (PMDD) that is a result of hormonal changes that take place in the months prior to menstrual cycle and during the ovulation. As women enter the menopausal age becoming more vulnerable to depression and also bone loss as well as bone loss and osteoporosis. According to scientists the conditions are common with menopausal due to changes in estrogen levels and other hormones of women.

Women who suffer from depression may become more severe due to other factors like stress at work or at home. Women often have to balance their work and family obligations. They be at work, look after their children and perform household chores at once which makes them more vulnerable to the symptoms of depression. They are even more susceptible to developing the disorder in the event that they have issues with relationships and abuse.

Depression in Men

Men are more likely to handle depression in a different way than women. Many men are reluctant to discuss the condition since they consider it an indication of weakness. The result is that they be more vulnerable to problems over time. They also are more susceptible to commit suicide.

In the same way, men are likely to have different symptoms than women. For women, depression typically is accompanied by feelings of guilt, sadness and a sense of worthlessness. For men, depression typically is accompanied by exhaustion and irritability. People who are depressed are more likely to stop engaging in the activities that they were previously enjoying. They also are more likely to consume and abuse illicit drugs and alcohol.

Infections that are often co-existing with depression

There are diseases that typically occur prior to or during the beginning of depression. They're usually the root or effects to the condition. People suffering from depression must be aware of other conditions that are associated with it , so they are able to effectively manage the issue before it becomes worse.

Anxiety disorders like obsessive compulsive disorder(OCD), panic disorder and post-traumatic stress disorder generalized anxiety disorder and social phobia typically are associated with depression. For example, after having an event that is traumatic, such as an accident, someone might develop post-traumatic stress disorder and. However, people with chronic post-traumatic stress disorders are more likely to suffer from depression.

Based on a study conducted in collaboration with the National Institute of Mental Health More than 40% of people suffering from post-traumatic stress disorder experienced depression within four months following an traumatic experience.Likewise researchers have found that depression is more likely to coexist with alcohol or substance abuse, which can be a trigger for mood disorders. The study also revealed that depression can be co-occurring alongside other health conditions, such as cancers, diabetes and strokes, heart attacks, AIDS or HIV, and Parkinson's disease.

Patients who have depression as well as another medical condition are more likely to experience greater severity of symptoms, and have greater difficulty in managing their illness. They also face higher costs. But, they should be advised to treat co-occurring illness to alleviate the symptoms that are associated with depression.

The various Types of Depression

Knowing the various kinds of depression can help you recognize the severity of your illness and the best treatment options.

Major Depressive Disorder, also known as Major Depression. This kind of depression manifests itself as the combination of symptoms that can interfere on the capability to rest or eat, work, study, and perform normally. It could be debilitating in the event that it is not treated promptly. Someone suffering from major depression disorder could have a single episode or several episodes in the course of his life.

Dysthymia or Dysthymic Disorder. This kind of depression is characterised by chronic symptoms that are generally not severe, which means it's not debilitating. However, the symptoms are significant enough to keep people from functioning as they should at school, work or at home. They also have a negative impact on the rest of society. The person suffering from dysthymic disorder usually has symptoms that last at 2 years at a minimum. It is possible that they will have several episodes during his life.

Minor Depression. This kind of depression manifests itself through symptoms that don't meet the criteria of major depression. The symptoms are usually at least two weeks. Anyone suffering from minor depression must seek help as soon as he can. If not, the minor depression could turn into a major depression.

Psychotic Depression. This kind of depression can occur when depression gets excessive to the point that it can cause psychosis. The patient may experience delusions or false belief as well as hallucinations. They might be able to hear or see things that others can't be able to see or hear.

Postpartum Depression. Contrary to what is commonly believed postpartum depression can be much more severe than the baby blues. Baby blues happen when the body of women who just gave birth experience hormonal and physical changes. Women can also be overwhelmed by the new responsibility to care for their baby. Baby blues fade within a short time, however postpartum depression can last longer. According to research, 10 to 15 percentage of moms who had their babies have postpartum depression.

Seasonal Affective Disorder (SAD). This kind of depression is defined by the beginning of depression during the winter cold months. At this time of the year, the majority of people are outside. Therefore, many sufferers experience the seasonal disorder of affective disorders. But, when the season is changed and they see the sun begins to shine brightly the moods of people also shift and improve. As the spring and summer season arrive individuals' moods improve and their seasonal affective disorder goes away. The people who suffer from seasonal affective disorders may go through the psychotherapy of light and light. They could also use prescription medication , and then combine treatment.

Bipolar Disorder or Manic Depression. This kind of depression is characterised by maniatic episodes which change in conjunction as depression episodes progress. The people who suffer from this condition are more likely to experience intense mood fluctuations. Sometimes, they become extremely ambitious or enthusiastic, leading them to come up with crazy thoughts and plans for all kinds of things. However, after a while they start to become depressed and depressed.

Depression symptoms and signs

Patients suffering from depression also to experience a variety of symptoms. But there are many different symptoms that are identical for all people. For instance, your symptoms might not be identical to those of people you know who have similar symptoms. In addition, your frequency and intensity of your symptoms might be different depending on the condition you suffer from.

Here are the top frequently observed symptoms and signs of depression that are observed in the most patients suffering from the condition:

Anxiety, sadness and feelings of desperation

The feeling of hopelessness or despair

Inability to engage in pleasure or hobbies

A decrease in energy levels

Fatigue

It is difficult to recall details, taking choices, and keeping focus

Morning wakefulness, frequent sleeping or insomnia

Appetite loss

Overeating

Suicide-related attempts or thoughts of suicide

Aches or pains, cramps digestive issues, headaches that are not alleviated when treated with conventional treatments

The diagnosis of depression

Many sufferers of depression think that their situation will never improve. This is not accurate since even the most serious cases of depression are treatable. When you notice signs of depression then you must go to a physician. The earlier you begin treatment the faster you will recover.

The first step is visiting a mental health professional or doctor and have them perform check-ups and medical assessments. Note that certain illnesses and viruses could cause symptoms like depression. Therefore, it is important to conduct physical examinations as well as interviews and laboratory tests to confirm that you are not suffering from the conditions mentioned above. After these conditions are eliminated, you are able to begin the psychological assessment.

Your doctor may recommend you to a psychiatrist or mental health professional who will ask concerning your history with regard to your illness and the history of your family members with depression. Be sure to be truthful when you are evaluating. Do not be afraid to discuss your issues. Also, you should be able to explain what caused them and how long they've been present. Also, you should discuss the severity of their effects and the way they impact your daily life.

The doctor might ask whether your symptoms have been present prior to. If they did been, you must tell your doctor about how you were treated. The doctor can also inquire whether you have used alcohol or drugs or whether you've had thought of suicide, or even death. If you've been diagnosed with depression, you need to seek treatment right away.

Common causes of depression

According to studies that depression is caused by a mixture of genetic, biological psychological, chemical, social, and environmental elements. Depression is generally a sign of an unbalance in the mental, bodily, and emotional condition of the person. It could happen for no apparent reason .

Here are a few of the most frequently occurring reasons for depression that can be discovered in those suffering from the disorder:

Life events

Depression can occur due to traumatic or painful experiences, such as being attacked or beaten.

Loss

It is also possible for someone to develop depression following a significant loss, like the loss of the job they had, a beloved one, or even a home. People can also be depressed when they move from one stage in their lives to another, like moving from working to retirement.

Anger

Some people describe depression as frozen anger. This type of anger is typically expressed as depression when internally bottled up. It is usually the case when people feel powerless and angry and aren't able to communicate their feelings because of the fear of being judged or mocked.

Childhood experiences

Someone who has been emotionally or physically abused, have experienced traumatizing events in their childhood or did not manage to develop effective coping strategies as children tend to be depressed. They also struggle to deal with depression.

Physical physical

Depression could be caused by physical issues. It is, however, frequently overlooked by people who tend to focus on physical symptoms it brings. Here are a few of the physical disorders that can trigger depression:

The hormones are involved in a variety of issues, including thyroid and parathyroid issues

Low blood sugar levels

Menstrual symptoms that are associated with menopausal symptoms

Conditions that impact the brain and nervous system.

Sleep issues

If you are suffering from any of the ailments mentioned above, ensure it that you tell your physician so that these problems can be identified through blood tests. Remember that having depression is not an indication of weakness. Everyone, even the most strong people on earth is able to suffer from depression. Depression can be a severe mental condition that affects females and males regardless of race, age or social situation. It may be ongoing, chronic and short-lived or even long-lasting. It's also the leading reason for disability, in accordance with the World Health Organization. This is the reason you need to address your depression with a seriousness. You must find ways to beat it in the shortest possible time.

Chapter 2: Causes Of Depression

In the last chapter, we examined the many frequently asked questions on the subject and I responded to questions with the greatest of ability. The next chapter we'll be focusing on the root causes of depression, and help you to determine your own symptoms.

Personal reasons

Problems with relationships

Being in a relationship that is not working is thought to be among the main reasons for depression. It is possible to have partners who can be difficult to reconcile to; or who create emotional and mental trauma. People who are in this situation are more likely to suffer from depression as they may suffer from emotional, mental or physical pain in a day-to-day basis. This type of relationship may not necessarily be between couples but could include parents, their siblings, children, grandparents or even grandparents.

Health of your family

Personal health issues can lead individuals to suffer from depression and anxiety, without doubt. However, family health issues will result in anxiety. If it's an elder member of the family or older person they're suffering from health issues, it's likely that they will experience anxiety. They tend to over worried over their physical and mental wellbeing and, as a result, they will be pushed toward depression.

Responsibilities

Being burdened with a lot of responsibility that fall on your shoulders could result in depression. In the event that you've got a huge family to care for as well as numerous charges to settle, or take charge of elderly people, etc. Then you're bound to feel depressed. If you are under lots of pressure at work that is exacerbated by an uneasy relation with your partner, all of these factors will create a situation that will appear to be extremely difficult for you. You may begin to feel your depression, accompanied by anxiety attacks.

Physical causes

Hormonal imbalance

One of the main physical reasons for depression is hormone imbalance. This is particularly prevalent in women as their hormones are constantly fluctuating each month. Brain cells produce a substance called cortisol to help reduce stress. If the woman leads an uncontrollable lifestyle, this can further aggravate the situation , and she will just push herself further into depression.

Genetic disposition

It is believed that there are depression genes that could be passed down from parents to their children. Although there isn't any definitive proof of this but there have been tests conducted on children and parents who both reported being depressed. Researchers have discovered a link however they are not able to pinpoint the exact kind of gene that are passed on.

Childhood incident

In the event of a devastating childhood event, then being aware of it could lead to depression. Events like sexual assault, abuse or other violent act can lead to depression. Being addicted to smoking and taking drugs at an early age is thought to trigger people to become depressed because their hormones will be in a state of imbalance and their cortisol levels are high.

Injury

A head injury can lead to depression in the sufferer. If they are struck on the head and there is a minor injury in the area of the brain in which cortisol is normally produced, then the individual starts to be depressed. In the same way, if there's an increase in brain or there is a tumor then the individual will begin to experience depression.

Environmental issues

Pollution

The environmental factors like pollution are the main reason for people to experience depression. Pollution is a source of harmful chemicals that cause the body and mind of people to change. Pollution can also trigger physical ailments, which could result in depression. While the majority of pollution is caused by car emissions, some of the pollutants that are found in the air originate from factories, which could be more destructive.

Extreme weather

Extreme weather conditions, such as excessive heat or too many cold temperatures can make people feel anxious and can lead to depression. The extreme climate can cause bodies to experience pain. They may not be aware of it because the process are internal and insignificant. If someone is required to spend time in a sauna for the whole month, he or will likely be extremely uncomfortable and definitely suffer from depression. In the same way, if a person is forced to sit in a fridge, the person cannot be normal. There are nations that are prone to extreme weather conditions throughout the year. Moving to a place like that can result in depression.

Natural disasters

The fear of natural disasters can be depressing. In places where there is always the possibility of a natural disaster hitting, like the worry of a tsunami that occurs in a coastal region or the worry of a hurricane, individuals there could experience anxiety and be depressed. Being in a new place and experiencing a culture shock could be a trigger for people to develop anxiety as they come learn to blend in with the locals.

Social causes

Teasing

Being teased by other people and even eve teased could be cause of depression. A bully can make people fear what they may confront next , and they begin to worry and panic. This could trigger anxiety and can further lead to depression. Being teased by males and being forced to do things at your own will can cause depression, especially if there's no means by which the bullying or teaser is made to cease. It can happen almost anyplace, such as college, school office, home, and more.

Friendship issue

If you've experienced the loss of a close friend or someone that was near to you it's likely that people will begin to suffer from depression. The process of accepting the loss of a loved-one can be difficult and causes people to suffer anxiety and stress. It could be a relative, or the relative of a friend. Being faced with the loss of a loved one could be a huge burden on the mind, and can cause people to experience depression.

Peer pressure

Peer pressure can lead people to experience anxiety. Being a part of a group or attempting to be part of an environment can be difficult , and can cause individuals to develop anxiety. It can take time and lead people to suffer from depression. Certain friends may pressure you to try drinking, smoking, or similar bad habits that can cause people to spiral into a downward spiral and ultimately develop depression.

These are a few reasons , and if you recognize the cause which is causing depression, you may be able to try and lessen the type of depression you are experiencing using the methods described in chapter 4.

Chapter 3: Easing to Feel Awed

If a tiny baby opens their eyes and observes something for the first time, you will witness awe-inspiring wonder in the eyes of the child. As they grow older and discover more exciting experiences, that awe present. When we get too caught up with the material things of life and lose sight of the things that really amaze us. We may think that things are cool at times but that's not really the same as being in awe. Awe happens the moment you look around and experience a positive feeling of inspiration generated by the things you see or the surroundings. It's possible to bring that to your life from time to time and it's a good thing because, when you are in that state of awe, you're overwhelmed that you forget about all the troubles you've been facing. If you believe in the existence of God or Gods, you might feel closer to God because of your the most awe-inspiring of surroundings. Let me give you some examples of places people believe are incredible in the truest sense of the word:

The hill is located in countryside that is surrounded by views and sunset or sunrise

A beach that is empty at sunset/sunrise.

The mountain is high in the sky at sunset or sunrise

Looking out over a waterfall at sunrise or sunset

What is the reason for sunset or sunrise? The hues that are added to the scenery during these times are beautiful and can lift away from the monotony of everyday life to a world that is alive and well. This kind of setting can also make you feel small and possibly vulnerable, but in a good way. For instance, if you decide to relax by the water at sunset, you could be amazed by the beauty of the scene to you, but you may also be a bit tiny when compared to. The feeling of being closer to God or even the natural world is something worth holding to. Although you might see yourself as being as small like a grain of sand by comparison, you must to recognize that without you, in the picture there could be no beach, since those grains of sand could have no existence. Therefore even though you're tiny, you are essential to the entire picture you become a part of.

Breathing exercise - As you're in this spot that inspires you, ensure you are supported and you have a good posture. There's a solid reason behind this. The proper posture will allow for a greater energy flow in your body. Even if it's not your belief in things such as Chakras there is a good chance that you believe in acupuncture. In this particular medical practice needles are inserted into specific locations to facilitate the flow of energy. Straight sitting does the same thing, allowing you to put your body in a perfect posture to breathe properly and to feel well.

Inhale through the nose for seven seconds. Keep the breath in your mouth for a while before exhaling until you reach eight. When you inhale, ensure that it feels like the air is going down your stomach and you will start to feel a pivoting movement when you breathe properly. Continue to do this, and focus on breathing as you exhale and inhale.

Depressed people may turn their feelings into the dark side, affecting the level of oxygen in their blood due to being emotionally overwhelmed. This is the reason people experience panic attacks. While practicing this breathing exercise you're inhaling fresh air and making sure that you are in an extremely calm state which is essential for your well-being. You'll feel more energized and more energetic and this will help you fight depression.

Test your observational skills

See the world around you from this awe-inspiring place and try to remember every detail you can, including the colors you can see. Close the eyes, and attempt to imagine the scene in your head. Take note of the hues. Take note of the different architectural elements of the scene. Once you believe you've crafted an accurate picture of what you saw, you can open your eyes and check what you missed. Visualization is crucial to move on to the next chapter since you'll be able achieve goals by using visualization to stimulate you to do what you need to do. It also gives you an incentive, and this is often lacking when you're feeling suffering from depression. So, learn to create images within your head so that you are able to empower yourself.

If you're interested in testing yourself once more, ask someone to place lots of inspirational things around the room in which you're sitting and observe. Put your head in a corner and attempt to explain to your companion what you observed. This can help you improve your ability to imagine. This will benefit you because visualization can help for escaping thoughts of despair. In the next section, you will be taught the use of visualization to help you feel more calm or calm when depression is taking over. This means that you're in a position to locate an escape path until the time of self-doubt is over. It's a great tool to avoid being in a depression.

Chapter 4: The Inside On Positivity

Before discussing positivity or positive emotions, it's essential to understand the relationship between its antagonist , negative thoughts and depression.Here's the fact: depression is the result of negative thoughts, feelings, as well as feelings.Those are the materials that can ignite through which the flame of depression may be stoked further more.Therefore being a perpetual pessimist is an assured way to remain depressed or, worse, getting more depressed.

If you're depressed how would it feel when your most trusted friend says to you "Wow you're depressed? I've discovered that clinical depression is practically an all-time sentence for an existence of doom and despair! You need to prepare yourself to be ready for this! "Chances are that you'll feel even more helpless, hopeless and depressed! That's the point where optimism or a positive attitude can be a factor.

How do you define Positivity?

Positivity refers to a belief or approach to thinking that focuses on the positive aspects of things.Positivity does not imply - contrary to what many naive "realists" believe exaggerating the positives, and denial or minimizing the negative aspects of life.Having an optimistic attitude is believing that things will eventually work out for positive, even if the situation is difficult right now.

Why is positivity important, especially when you're experiencing clinical depression?Positivity has physical and mental benefits.Some of the physical benefits of having a generally positive attitude include:

- A longer life;

- Greater ability to handle the stress of everyday life;

- Healthier blood pressure;

- Greater tolerance to physical or other types of pain;

Improved physical health

- Lower risk of heart issues; and

- Stronger immune system.

Positive mental health advantages are:

- Greater ability to handle;

Improved capability to solve issues;

Creativity is increased;

- Improved mental clarity

- Lighter mood;

Better management for depression e.g. feelings less depression.

Hope for Pessimists

The idea of being positive is an desirable attitude to have.But not all people are naturally optimistic as well as optimistic.Many people, which could include you, have been through life's challenges that have conditioned their minds to be taught to believe that the worst will happen in order to shield themselves from more damaging experiences.If are a pessimist do you have the ability to develop an optimistic outlook on life?

There's good news and not-so-good-but-not-really-bad news.The good news is positivity is something that can be developed or acquired through consistent and intentional practice and is not an either-you-have-it-or-you-don't type of trait. The not-so-good-but-not-really-bad news is that if you're a pessimist, it will take effort and commitment to do so.It's not going to be a walk in the park.But as my relatively overweight friends who were able to train for and finish a full marathon would say, it's hard, but it's doable and is worth the hardship.

There's more to this idea or principle than fantasies thinking.One study of people who focused on positive and positive thoughts daily found that subjects started to feel more positive throughout the day, when they began the regular practice.Other studies have also demonstrated that positive thoughts can help sick and depressed patients deal with their ailments regardless of whether they view themselves as being naturally optimistic.

General Positivity Principles

Before you are able to be more positive It is important to conduct some mental cleaning first.How do you accomplish this? By checking your mind for any negative thoughts that are running through your mind, such as:

Poor Mental Filters: These are the mindsets that tend to make the negatives worse and ignore the positives.For instance, let's say that you're watching how the Golden State Warriors beat the Hell from The Houston Rockets in game 3 of the 2017-2018 NBA Western Conference Finals series in an epic 41-point win.Let's imagine that your most beloved star is Zaza Pachulia, who's barely played in the playoffs.A poor mental filter can be complaining about the "dumb" Steve Kerr is for not playing your favorite Zaza in that game. To the point that you're not even concerned that the Warriors have handed the Rockets the most brutal playoff loss in the history of their franchise!

- Blame-Taking:This is a mindset that may appear to be "responsible" or pro-active, but is actually an extreme and mentally unhealthy version of taking responsibility.Blame-taking is a pessimist mental filter because the person feels he or she's inadequate or always at fault for everything that goes wrong in the world - including the abrupt cancellation of the hit U.S. T.V. series Designated Survivor!

The concept of disaster anticipation is an internal filter that causes you to expect the worst to happen in any circumstance you're in.For instance, you're out of coffee and didn't get the morning cup of Joe prior to leaving for work . You feel that it's a sign for even worse things to come such as the lack of coffee at work, or the fact that you boss might actually offer you some advice!

Extreme Thinking: This refers to the tendency to view things solely as pure white or black, without any shade of gray between.With this kind of mental filter it is either perfect or deplorable.

If you can find the filters that you've been looking for within your head then the next step is to acknowledge them, quickly let them go, and then shift your attention to the positive aspects about the situation or circumstance you're facing.And by focussing on the positive aspects I'm not suggesting that you sweep negative issues that must be put beneath the rug.What I'm recommending here is to concentrate your mental and physical focus on the positives i.e. the things that can be accomplished instead of what isn't able to be done, how situations can be improved rather than the reasons why they can't be changed and the best way to deal with issues instead of focusing on what the difficulties are.Think with a clear mind and make sure that people are responsible for what they do in the future after you've dealt with the situation.

As I mentioned earlier, establishing an optimistic attitude can require time, especially in the case of those who are naturally pessimistic.But with perseverance positive thinking can be an automatic habit that's naturally to you.

Chapter 5: Food And Exercise

Food

It is likely that you have eaten all kinds of unhealthy things. It's tempting to consume foods with a lot of sugar to gain energy when you're depressed. But, the exercises you engage in will result in the same. Exercise is a source of energy by itself. So, keep in mind that fruits are your primary source of sugar. If you're overweight, this can lead to depression, as you might have issues with how you appear. Do not cut back on food. A diet won't benefit you in the least. Change the foods you eat to have a wide diverse.

I noticed that the replacement food made a huge difference. Amount of bread I consumed was limited but not banned. The issue when you're depression is that it makes you are prone to think of everything as white and black, and it's not. There are gray areas too. Replace butter with Omega spreads that are based on

Omega; eat foods high in Omega like fish since they help keep brain cells active. Reduce your intake of sugary food you consume and try not to eat too much at night. It's not the right time for food deprivation. It's the time to be sensible. I was aware that chocolates make me fat, but I did allow myself to have a couple of chocolates each day, and they were delicious, instead of eating a complete box at once. It's true that when you restrict your consumption instead of eating a lot or eating a large amount, you appreciate food a lot more.

When you sit at the table for a meal it is not a good idea to let yourself become an uninvolved eater. Create a feasting ritual and place the table. Your posture while sitting to eat needs to be straight, as it assists digestion. If you're not able to consume everything, don't worry about it. Make an effort to consume a wide range of food especially those that are high with Omega 3 because these really can help you gain the strength. If you're unable to put it all together to cook fantastic foods like fish, you should consider Omega 3 supplements because they actually help with depression.

Exercise

Everyone is apprehensive at the thought of exercising, particularly when they're feeling depressed. The thought of getting out the door in the morning was a source of anxiety for me. Introduce it gradually. Go into the nearby shop to purchase a daily paper. The walk will allow you begin to be awed by the fresh air. If you're not well-behaved, having a dog can help since it will give you something you can be concerned about that's not yours. People with depression tend to think about others more than they think of themselves. If you need to exercise your dog, it will give you an incentive to exercising.

Another activity you could accomplish is to perform one small task. Your home may need it. I can remember gazing at everything that was settling within my rooms. It was an awful sight. Most likely, you're not conscious about it. However, you should make you aware. It's not necessary to tackle everything at once. Clean the furniture and watch it shine. This is how your life is going to shine in the coming years. Just get your head around it. You will be surprised that just a tiny piece of cleaning each moment will soon bring your home to a spick and clear and you'll feel more at ease in your home.

Mixing exercise with Meditation

It's likely that it has never thought of that you might be depressed, there's a good chance you're thinking negative thoughts. If you are able to take a stroll in the local park and focus on the positive things in the surrounding area even for the brief duration you're sitting It's a fantastic mental exercise. Meditation isn't just about thinking about nothing. It could mean thinking about anything and everything, but not the root of your troubles. In this situation you have to discipline yourself not to dwell on your depression. Instead, be in a calm place and absorb all the things nature will show you. Take a look at the flowers coming into bloom. See kids running around the park. Be amazed by the way clouds alter their shape.

There's a lot to see and you don't have to put in a lot of effort to accomplish that. Find a comfy park bench or a bench near the ocean and relax and observe the world move around you. It doesn't require physical effort. It's about mental energy and it is essential for this part of yourself in order to get back into the flow of the world, to look at things and to appreciate all the wonderful things that happen in the world. The blueness of the ocean as well as the green of the gardens and the various shades of the sky. They all exist to heal you. I remember lying on my the bed, looking up at the clouds and noticing various shapes in them. There were faces, and other objects like babies, and even trees. Take note and let your experience be positive, because there is plenty of beauty in the world and you can take part of it by finding a spot in which you can take a seat and admire it.

When you're doing this, make sure you breathe in a controlled manner, since anxiety is common for those who suffer from depression. If you are able to conquer anxiety by breathing in particular manner, it will be easy to decrease anxiety. Breathe through your nose and count to five as you keep your breath. Be focused on your breathing. Let the air go escape your body. However, be aware of the air entering your body and then leaving it. Try to exhale more air than you breathe in. There's a reason behind this. People who panic tend to panic due to the fact that they take in air or hyperventilate. It is possible to do breathing exercises any time during the day. You just need to integrate them into your daily routine.

Keep in mind that word "routine. There may not be one in the present however, we must bring you to a point where you do regardless of whether it's executed in auto mode for now. The reason why this routine is so crucial is that without it, you're not able look around your surroundings or think about any thing. It's uncomfortable to be looking towards scrubbing your carpet and then scrubbing it again, but I did it and you'll be amazed at how wonderful it felt to do it. I used a nail brush and made circular movements on the rug that was dirty . All of the shades came out to me, colors I had not seen for a long time. It was an act of love however once you begin to see the results of your work you'll see the reason why I tell you that you must have one.

The problem comes when you are off the path of life and realize that depression is keeping you from doing things that cause issues with. It's likely that's what you're experiencing right today. Select a little item - from your routine list. It's not difficult to integrate it into your routine. First, you must make is to differentiate between night and day and realize that each serves a purpose.If you're having trouble sleeping the energy levels of your body are low, but you are the only one to get you back on track. I'm going to show you how by utilizing my own experiences and I am aware of how difficult it can be. You're not feeling like doing all of these things However, what you're doing is sending yourself back in the world, saying "Hey you must be careful - I'm back."

Although nobody is aware that you have did your best to clean your teeth, you are aware. You're feeling more clean, your skin feels fresher and you feel as if you're getting somewhere. Everyone doesn't notice when washing your face, except yourself and it awakens the various nerve endings that are present and can be quite alarming whenever you've not done it for a long time. This stimulation is deliberate and your method of getting out of the chrysalis and becoming a human after a time of depression.

Relaxation Exercise

It's really simple. The only thing that you are allowed to focus on is the portion of your body you're focusing at and breathing. There is nothing else you can think about. If you are lying on your bed in a calm space and block out all interruption, you must breathe in a controlled manner. Shut your eyes, and begin using your toes. Tensify them until you're aware Then, allow them to relax completely. They'll appear weighty. Try this on all of your body, from your thighs to your temples. Finally, let yourself relax your eyes slowly and gradually be aware of the space is yours before you leave bed and begin your day. This is an exercise that energizes you, however, it also helps you to enter an extremely relaxed state, and that is what you require. Treat yourself to a treat every day. It's also a great spot to go to when problems are causing you to feel upset. You can simply excuse yourself and take a relaxing exercise, and you'll get more energy out of it.

The workout you're providing yourself with is mental fitness in addition to physical and both can help overcome depression. The reason this works is because your breathing can help you feel more relaxed. You won't be stressed or agitated since you'll be more calm. You'll be able to accept things that you could not before. You can listen to your music of choice. Do not listen to music that has made you unhappy that you've heard in the past. It's a source of depression. Instead, choose to listen to something that lifts you up.

I'm not a typical opera lover However, listening to some songs in the Cavaliera Rusticana was a great way to feel so incredibly emotionally that the songs made me stop in my tracks by their beautiful beauty. I needed to sit and meditate on the music for a while. That's okay. I've also experienced moods when I was listening to the music of the sixties and then jumped around trying for a dance. It's fine. Anything that is energizing every part of your mind or body is good, so let yourself indulge in a bit. The goal is to bring your senses back to life after having been slowed by depression , because that's the aspect of your life that which you do not think about. It's there. Your emotions are positive, and regardless of the circumstances, you are an extremely vital human being.

It was one piece music that truly lifted my spirits. It was known as a concerto for two voices. I would listen to it to inspire me. I never thought that the two voices would sound this great. I don't usually like barbershop type music however this was entirely different. There were other pieces that I loved playing on the classical guitar, but I did not stop there. I also listened to some fantastic electric guitar too. Whatever is your favorite is the perfect music to complete your tasks to. Still in depression which means you go through fluctuations, but when you utilize music to bring your mood to a more positive level, it can be effective. Consider:

Which song lifts me up?

* What songs make me smile?

* Which song makes me feel beautiful?

* What songs make me dance?

Each of these is a important tools to have currently since you can alter your mood by yourself. If you are contemplating things that make you feel depressed, you, play music that helps you relax. If you are feeling down choose music that brings you joy. My happy music was composed from an French composer Erik Satie because he's the only person I've met who could make the sound of the piano as if it's singing rather than simply being a music instrument. It's different for you due to the fact that you're an individual, but whatever you do allow yourself the moments of happiness.

Chapter 6: Your Strength Of Exercise And Your Body!

It was stated in the previous article that the imbalance of chemicals within the brain can cause depression. But, we can alter the brain's chemistry in a significant way without medications! The most simple and enjoyable method to do this is to exercise.

If you exercise your brain produces an endorphin-like chemical, that is known as the endorphins. Regular exercise improves the balance of chemicals within the brain. This is why it is the most effective natural treatment for depression. It's also enjoyable as well!

Yes, fun! It is possible that you are not the kind of person who likes exercising, or perhaps you were a regular exerciser but because of depression, you've lost interest. This chapter is focused on providing you with a fun exercise that you'll take pleasure in and that is easy to master.

Exercise is believed to be the most effective treatment for mild and moderate depression. It also aids in the treatment of those suffering from severe depression. According to research regular exercise can help alleviate symptoms of anxiety and depression. A regular exercise routine can decrease stress, enhance sleep quality and boost confidence in yourself. It's a wonderful combination of benefits!

As mentioned earlier as we have discussed earlier, your body releases endorphins after exercising. Endorphins are extremely powerful chemical compounds. They are amazing"feel great" chemicals are able to interact with receptors that are located in your brain. This can decrease the perception of pain. Endorphins work as analgesics. You can get a small "high" during exercising!

Endorphins create a positive emotion within your body. There is a tendency to feel happy after exercising. This is commonly referred to as "runner's feeling". Imagine yourself now being euphoric and experiencing the opposite of depression! Feeling joy, happiness, delight and deep joy! It's similar as the drug morphine. But, unlike morphine endorphins aren't addictive.

Exercise is among the most effective treatment options for depression. In addition to helping you conquer depression, regular exercise will also bring these advantages:

Your heart is strengthened and can prevent the development of heart disease.

Lowers blood pressure

It helps reduce the stress-inducing agent known as cortisol in your brain.

Your body is strengthened while increasing the tone of your muscles

Aids in losing excess weight, and also reduce the body's fat.

It makes you look healthier and healthy

Training will help you look and feel great. It's an easy cheap, cost-effective and scientifically-proven treatment for depression. Any type of exercise can aid in easing depression. These are just a few of the fun activities you can incorporate into your exercise routine to help stop or treat depression:

Dancing

Dancing can be a fun method to let all the blues off! Dancing can help you get fit. Additionally, it has lots of other advantages. It's a fun activity which can also help reduce stress. Try:

Zumba

Belly dancing

Ballroom dancing

Ballet

Hip-hop

Dancing is an excellent pastime. It's also a cheap method to combat depression because you do not require any equipment. It also improves your endurance, flexibility and strength. Also, it comes with the benefit of being extremely social and social. You may meet wonderful people there. If the thought of that is a bit daunting at the moment Don't be worried. Dance in your living room with some fantastic music! It may seem silly at first, but time being foolish can be very great for us!

Biking

If you're the athletic kind You can also try biking. Biking can be fun too. You will see beautiful scenery as you travel. Explore the outdoors and create a more enjoyable experience!

Golf

Golf is an excellent exercise option, particularly in the event that you decide to walk instead of riding the cart. It's also a fantastic method to make connections with your fellow golfers. The connection with nature as well as the education involved will make you feel relaxed and rejuvenated.

Mixed Martial Arts

Many fitness enthusiasts want to take on mixed martial art. It's considered to be among the most sought-after types of training. If you're looking to build your strength, endurance and self-defense abilities, then this exercise is the one for you. It is a great movement, so your body can release plenty of endorphins during one workout. It is an challenging form of exercise however the joy and knowledge that it brings will completely change your self-image and there's no release of endorphins as powerful!

Housework

There is no have to employ the services of a housekeeper or cleaner. Housework is among the most efficient methods to keep active and beat depression. Make sure you sweep or mop your floors every day. Cleansing your home is an excellent method of releasing all the endorphins!

Does this sound like a nightmare? Do a little task at home and then an hour later, you'll see you've completed a lot! It's because it becomes addicted and releases dopamine within the brain. We'll get to that later.

Tennis

Tennis is a great sport and provides excellent exercise for all the parts of your bodytoo. It is easy to feel relaxed after a successful sport! Enjoy the sun in the outdoors to increase your happiness!

Walking

Walking is a gentle exercise that will help you feel better immediately. Walking will make you feel at ease. It's particularly beneficial when you're worried, stressed and stressed. Go for a walk in the countryside or walk with a companion or meditate as you walk! Be aware and present of the surrounding environment including the sky, the earth your breath, and your feet. Walking on a regular basis can be an amazing experience when we are completely present.

Yoga

Yoga is among the most effective exercises you can do in times of depression. Yoga allows you to stay in touch to your body. In times of depression, we tend to get caught up in our thoughts over and over, immersed by thoughts, and completely away from the world around us as well as other people as well as our own bodies. Yoga can help you get more grounded. By practicing regularly, it will allow you to manage your emotions more effectively. Attend a class for social benefits as well!

If you're experiencing depression, you require a an emotional and social support system that is strong. It is therefore recommended to take part in a class with a group. You can make your workouts more enjoyable by working out with your family and fellow gym members. If you participate in this way, you will benefit not just from your physical workout but also from the emotional support that you receive from your family and friends. There is no need to join an instructor-led class even if it doesn't interest you, however. Just get moving!

There is no need to perform all of these exercises If you'd rather another type of exercise you can do it! Maybe you like the flowing, slow moves of tai chi or the adrenaline thrill of heli-skiing in the Swiss Alps or the simple feeling of in the green fields of your buddies and the waves crashing against your kite surfing or the incredible hypertrophy that comes from the last time you did your best of bodybuilding exercises, or even the exhilarating excitement of getting your wingsuit before you glide over the rock face. The key is to do whatever makes you happy!

Right now, I can see that a portion of you feels demotivated and doesn't want to leave the sofa, much less get up to the gym. This is why we can motivate ourselves and start working on it! Consider the tiniest easiest, most fun and simple baby step that you can take. When you are ready you, do the baby step. One thing can lead to another. It will be easier to make the next move.

Dopamine is which is the brain's "motivation chemical" is absent from the brain in people suffering from depression. However, the good news is dopamine is produced and released into the brain as we progress and achieve more. Therefore, the smaller actions we take the more dopamine gets release and how stimulated we feel! This is a cycle of good and bad. Consider that baby step, and make it the most simple and enjoyable manner the earliest you can!

It's not just exercise that makes you feel immediately better. You can utilize your body in a different way to feel better. Studies have found that laughter and smiles releases serotonin ("the happy chemical") in large amounts. Therefore, here's our next short easy, enjoyable, and fun activity.

1. It's probably the best thing to complete by yourself as you might appear strange!

2. Stand up elegant and tall, straight and without slouching a bit.

3. Take a look.

4. Smile wide from ear-to-ear. Smile!

5. Get laughing, laughing and laughing. Play a hilarious film or YouTube video or recall the most hilarious moment of your own life.

6. Get excited! Imagine that your depression has gone and your life has changed in the right direction! Imagine all the wonderful possibilities that could happen and all the small things to be thankful for. The more you practice this exercise the more this becomes a reality within your life!

Note that this exercise should be done after you have mastered the exercise in chapter 1. It is essential to be aware of your emotions and be aware of the impact they have on how you feel via your body's physiology. After you've mastered you emotional intelligence you'll feel free to practice this technique repeatedly and as long as you want. It's an absolute pleasure!

Chapter 7: The Body's Health:

Keeping It In Form

Many people consider happiness to be an inner sense of well-being which is a result of a balanced disposition in the mind and heart. But, a significant element of happiness is been linked to your physical fitness. In actual there have been numerous studies done to determine the connection of a healthy body to happiness and the findings have revealed the obvious: your odds of being happy and satisfaction are greater if do not suffer from any type of illness.

The findings of these studies have confirmed the essential importance of having an active lifestyle for alleviating any negative feelings you might be experiencing. Indeed, exercising in the treatment of certain ailments like depression has been proven to be extremely effective, with the rate of relapse being significantly lower than typical treatment for depression.

Here are the many ways in which physical exercise can create positive feelings of happiness and positivity:

Regularly exercise. There are numerous benefits for taking time each day or every week to exercise. You not only get to build strength and endurance as time passes, but you gain a positive perception about your physique. Additionally, you put yourself in a better position to feel happier and fulfilled. Researchers have discovered that those who exercise for 20 minutes experience greater levels of proteins and endorphins within the brain in comparison to people who remain in a stationary position for the same period. Endorphins, it is important to not forgotten, are neurotransmitters commonly believed by scientists to be those responsible for happiness. The higher the amount of endorphins released in the brainarea, the more satisfied you feel.

Take part in other physical actions, like dancing or sports. Engaging in a sport or thing you're interested in allows you to unwind and take a needed break from the stresses of daily life. It gives you the chance to stretch and become physically fit. It can even provide a therapeutic experience for others. Additionally, participating in team sports or other community sporting events is an effective way to promote the camaraderie of a group and increasing its general sense of happiness.

Get a good night's sleep. Much of how you'll feel throughout the day depends upon the level of the sleep you've had that previous night. If you awake with a wrong position bed, the chance of feeling irritable or, even more so, angry is increased. The feeling of anger and anger usually creates a ripple impact, meaning that other people you come into contact with will have to contend with the negative vibe that you emit, and could be irritated by it. It is essential to ensure that you get a restful night's rest which allows you to sleep completely and reenergized to tackle the challenges ahead.

Be mindful of your diet. A lot of people overlook the effects of food on their overall health and happiness. But it's important to recognize that your choices regarding food affect the way you feel. When deciding what foods to take in, it's better to focus on eating healthy foods that leave you feeling good about your self. Avoid processed foods as well as other choices that could result in cardiovascular and diabetes as well as other. This means that you should be extra cautious when choosing the food items you consume because in the future the choices you make now will be reflected in the near future. Also take note of the quantity of food you consume. Always eat in moderation any excess consumption will have negative results for the body and could affect your personal happiness.

Happiness is a decision, as they say and your life should reflect this. Take care of your physical health and wellbeing by taking good care of your body with exercising and a healthy diet. Make a conscious decision to feel happy by being healthy.

Chapter 8: Search of A Lifelong Happiness

The quest for satisfaction has always been the long-term goal for many, whether it be recognized in a conscious way or not. It was even mentioned within the Declaration of Independence of United States as a right granted to everyone by God.

The culture we live in advises us to seek success, fame, wealth and other material possessions in order to be content. The majority of us have taken that advice advice to heart and pursued these things in order to achieve happiness. Today we tend to are thinking of things they'd like to achieve to feel happy. People are more focused on the things they don't have instead of the things they do have, which can trigger feelings of anger, frustration and disappointment. In the course of our journey, we've lost sight of the reason for the pursuit and have instead concentrated on the external things.What people aren't aware of is that the desires of this world can be temporary ways to feel content. True happiness is derived from inside ourselves and not from the purchase of things aren't ours.

The wrong ideas about how to live a happy life have been formulated for quite a while, which were believed to be the most effective ways to be happy. Here are some examples.

Money can bring happiness. It is essential for daily life. Without it, you're unable to purchase basic necessities like shelter, food and clothing. However, many believe that accumulating an enormous fortune will be a source of happiness since you can purchase everything you'd like. For those who have the fortune of a lifetime anxiety and fear of losing money usually takes the place of the joy.

A relationship is going to make you feel happy. As mentioned above happiness is a result of within.Your happiness isn't dependent on the other people around you. While being with someone may make you feel happy but it is your personal decision to be content in any situation you happen to be in. Singles aren't in a bind if they have supportive and supportive family and friends who don't make you feel isolated. People who are single and engaged in worthwhile and successful endeavors that give them a sense of satisfaction are generally happier than those in unhappy relationships.

Happiness diminishes as you get older. It is likely that you have more responsibilities at the age of 65, however, that doesn't mean you're not more content than in your younger years. Since you are able to do more when you get older Your achievements bring joy for your existence. You can explore more of the world around you and pursue the things you enjoy. It has been proven that people who are older are happier and more content than middle and younger age adults. They are also more calm, stable emotionally and are less likely to experience negative emotions.

This is possibly because they've reached their goals in life, learned through their experiences, and are thankful to have reached that point.

Do you know of people who seem happier and more content than you? Are you depressed and believe that you won't be as content in the same way as them? Despair not. You can do about it. You can live as happily as the majority of people are, or even happier so long as you maintain the right attitude and mindset toward others, yourself and your situation. There isn't a magic formula in the art of achieving lifetime of happiness. What do those who are always content have in the common?

Be more positive

We are accustomed to discussing the negative aspects of our lives. This is evident in the newspapers and newscasts on television. The majority of articles or headlines focus on negative events such as murders, corruption or accidents. Negative thoughts can cause anxiety on us and cause unhappy.

It is said the universe attracts what you believe Therefore, train your brain to see the positive in every circumstance. Look for the positive in all things and believe that positive things will happen.Even negative situations can be a source of positive lessons. Reviewing the lessons you've learned will make you feel happier.

Always be thankful.

Research suggests that gratitude, as well as is a way to feel happy. It also promotes positive emotions and makes you feel confident about yourself. It also enhances your relationships with others.

Think about the things you are grateful for. Consider the experiences, people, and experiences that added significance in your daily life. Consider your blessings even the smallest of them. Thank God for another day and your food choices and for the people who appreciate and encourage you or the opportunities you have. Thank and praise those who do you an favor.

Develop meaningful relationships.

Man is not an is an island. Being connected to family, friends and special people or the communities is one of the most satisfying source of joy. You'll see that happy people generally have a good circle of family and friends that provide continuous encouragement and affection.

Keep your connections strong. Try to stay in touch with loved ones, despite your commitments or hectic schedule. Take time to spend time with them. Enjoy having the company of loved ones and talk to them about the things you're feeling or experiencing. Also, listen to what they share. This will strengthen your relationship.

You are who the people who you are hanging out with. Since happiness is infectious look for to be in the company of happy people. Their way of life will influence you , and you'll soon be just as happy as they are.

Take part in the happiness of other people. If you are enthusiastic and are interested in the positive luck of others you will be able to share their happiness too.

Joie de vivre

Live life to the fullest and enjoy the present moment. Keep your eyes and mind at the present. Don't dwell in the past and thinking about the future, because you'll be missing out on the positive things taking place all around you. If you let positive events go by without notice, they'll result in regrets, and you'll be tempted to dwell on these events again. This can create an endless cycle that can result in discontent and sadness.

Make time to feel the breeze against your face, take a moment to smell at the blossoms of your yard, feel the breath, or take in the food you're eating. These daily routines allow you to be conscious and enjoy moments of happiness in your life. Create daily routines that make you feel happy, such as going for a walk in the park each afternoon. You should concentrate on just one thing at a moment to take in the moment. You will not be able to enjoy your meal when you dine while watching TV. If you focus your complete concentration to just one thing, you'll be able to enjoy the most.

Have a good time!

It's real when they say that laughter is the most effective treatment. When you smile you release endorphins which help you feel in an enjoyable mood. The joy of laughter and humor can trigger happiness and helps ease your burdens anxiety or pain. And the best part about it is that it's completely free!

Give back and live your life with the meaning.

If you take part in rewarding activities, your self-esteem is more. It's because you believe that you have made an impact on the lives of other people. Volunteer at charity events , or more simply do actions of kindness. Make yourself more compassionate and generous. Discover your strengths and then join or start events that make use of them to benefit the entire community.

Exercise regularly.

A half hour of exercise is not only beneficial for your body, but it also benefits the mind, as it eases anxiety and stress. Pick a sport or an exercise that you are interested in and that you enjoy.

Get a good night's rest

A person should get 7 to 9 hours of rest each day. People are more prone to stress when you're not sleeping. It is also difficult to concentrate and think clearly.

Act

One of the causes of having depression is not being able to fulfill your desires or expectations that are not met. The negative thoughts of "I wish to...but I'm not able to", "What will happen" or "Maybe I'm going to lose" take over us. To stay clear of these thoughts, focus on the things you can accomplish. If you're planning to travel, and save money, get your backpack and get on the road. If you're looking for work prepare your resume and begin applying. Make sure you highlight the things you are good at. You're blessed with legs and hands and you can hike unlike disabled people who aren't able to. Transform your goals into achievable goals that guide your thoughts and boosts your energy levels. It also inspires your dreams. You'll then be content.

Select your response

In our daily lives there is always 90 90% response and 10% fate. In spite of the difficult circumstances If you decide to be positive, you'll enjoy your life today as well as tomorrow and for the rest of your life.

Chapter 9: What Harms Can Depression Cause?

We all experience sadness during those difficult moments in our lives, but it is usually gone after a certain period of time. But, when someone suffers from depression certain thoughts are self-destructing and potentially dangerous.

If depressive symptoms are not dealt with or treated properly it could direction toward:

Self-injury: Individuals who are depressed, and suffering from depression, may attempt to injure themselves. They may cut or burn themselves to temporarily relieve their depression. Sometimes, things can go out of hand and result in a fatal accident, or even the loss of life.

Suicide: When depression becomes more severe or isn't addressed in a timely manner, the person who is suffering could even commit suicide. In the midst of their despair they seek an escape from their pain and are often contemplating suicide as a means to get rid of the pain. If no one is looking at them during this time of stress or in the midst of a crisis and commit suicide.

Insane Actions: Because depression doesn't cause a person to have a plan for the future of their life, they typically engage in many dangerous activities, like driving drunk, speeding, inviting an uninvolved person home, or leaving alone at night in a risky neighborhood.

Health Risks A majority times, when someone is depressed people tend to quit sleeping and eating. In certain instances people overeat and then are more likely to be in sleeping. Additionally, they may occasionally become dependent on alcohol, sleeping pills or smoking. If depression-related episodes last for a prolonged period of time, these interruptions to a person's routine may cause grave damage to their health.

Insanity in Life Depression can result in lower performance in school or at work, as well being a source of issues in family relationships and life. Depression sufferers tend to be alone and are unable to respond to the concerns and questions of their family members. They become distracted from the work that is in front of them and are unable to focus on things. Their education, career and relationships could be affected to a large extent.

The effects of depression, you see, can trigger hazardous situations if it's serious and not addressed on time. In many instances, those suffering from depression are known to suffer for long periods of melancholy their mental equilibrium and attempt to commit suicide.

Although many describe depression as a temporarily sad or refer to the term 'feeling down' it is actually a major issue that can severely affect individuals. It is crucial to educate everyone about depression, particularly the those who are suffering from it or who have witnessed their loved ones suffering from it as well as methods to combat depression before it becomes severe, and that's the subject we'll be discussing during the following chapter.

Chapter 10: Different Types Of Depression

There are many causes of depression. Also, there are various types of depression which vary in severity and intensity of condition. It is crucial to know the type of depression as treatment or correction of the type of depression can also differ.

These are a few types of depression:

Major Depressive Disorder or Major DepressionThe kind of depression is characterised by a set of symptoms that impact and affects an individual's daily life (from eating, sleeping or working, and many more). The condition prevents the person from performing their duties normal. If you feel generally depressed or throughout the majority of the week, and are showing the typical signs of depression such as lack of enthusiasm for things you were once interested in and weight gain or loss and low energy levels, thoughts of suicide and many more it is possible to have been diagnosed as having Major Depression Disorder. Be aware that some people might suffer from a single episode throughout their lifetime, but typically it can happen repeatedly.

Persistent Depression Disorder - previously called dysthymia, persistent Depressive Disorder happens the case when a person's depression is believed to been present for two years or longer. But, the symptoms aren't so severe to disrupt day to everyday life, but it could hinder an individual's ability to effectively function and behave normally. A person diagnosed with Persistent Depressive Disorder might also experience an episode or a few periods that are a result of Major Depression.

Bipolar DisorderThis condition is typically marked as extreme mood swings with periods of energy that are high as well as periods that are low in energy. When there is a period that are low in energy individuals may exhibit symptoms associated with Major Depression. The use of lithium-based medications is commonly used to help stabilize mood.

Minor Depression - if an person is showing symptoms and signs of depression for a period of two weeks or more, but does not completely meet the criteria to be considered Major Depression, then he/she is likely to fall in the category of Minor Depression. However, it is crucial to remember that when Minor Depression is not treated it is a good chance that it could become a full-blown Major Depression Disorder.

There are different types of depression that have special circumstances like:

Seasonal Affective disorder - Major Depression in SAD often occurs during winter. The dark effect of shorter daylight hours and the fewer days.

Postpartum DepressionIt is likely that you've seen or heard about mothers who harm their infant child. One probable reason could be postpartum Depression. A majority of women experience this disorder following childbirth. This is evident in women who suffer from major depression in the following months or weeks after the birth of their child. It's not typical "baby blues" It's because of the mix of hormonal and physical changes, which are added to the parental responsibility and can become difficult to cope with.

Premenstrual Dysphoric Disorder (PMDD) is a second cause of hormonal imbalances/changes for women. Women suffering with PMDD may experience depressive episodes prior to the beginning menstrual cycle. In addition to depression, she could also experience irritation or irritability anxiety, fatigue and mood swings, changes in her eating and sleeping routines and difficulties in concentrating.

Psychotic Depression: this type of depression is particularly alarming due to the fact that an individual is facing an extreme depression with a form of psychosis. For instance, visions (seeing and hearing sounds that's not actually happening) and the feeling of paranoia (the belief that someone is trying to harm your feelings or make negative remarks regarding you) and illusions (false beliefs that break away from reality).

Different forms of depression require various forms of treatment and medications. One positive aspect can be that in even the most serious instances, depression can be efficiently treated, especially when symptoms are detected early on.

Chapter 11: Live For Entertainment

Sometimes, it's just a matter of wanting to be a vegetarian. Everyone does. It's important to take a break and do nothing at the time. Don't be afraid to feel like you're failing when you require to take a break.

Films

We all enjoy being entertained. Films allow us to escape from our personal world and immerse ourselves in the world of another. We can live the world from our screens. We can travel through time as well as space, and witness things that we would never be able to experience in reality. The movies are amazing. There are those who would keep watching to see what new movies are coming up with the next. What are the next plot concepts and the latest effects and changes to the makeup? What do your favorite stars are doing now? Films are available in a variety of styles; there's something for everyone. Are you wishing you could have more fun?

Take a look at a few comedy films from your favorite video retailer. Do you want to feel like you're experiencing the same things as you do? Go through Netflix and find a show that focuses on someone else who is experiencing the same thing. Are you willing to watch an hour of crappy entertainment? Go to the closest Redbox to rent the most groovy B-movie horror you will discover. The possibilities are endless. You could even revisit the past to discover the movies you enjoyed as a child and the ones that you watched repeatedly until you ran the tape and damaged the sound. Go through The Wizard of Oz 15 times per day if that's the thing you have to do to provide you with a reason to exist on this earth. Enjoy these classic movies with the younger generation. Take them to the cinema with your kids.

Books

Films, as well as books, are designed to help us escape. This is their primary reason for being. When you read an ebook and read, you don't only read but you also travel. You are enticed by the story, and are a part of the story through those characters. You can also be a young wizard or witch who flings wands and learns spells at your local wizarding school. It is possible to become werewolves. You can go to a world where children don't age and play games until the end of time. Fantasy is abounds in the pages of books. You are not limited to traveling to different times , but other worlds altogether. Spend some time for yourself, choose an area of peace in your home or at a your local bookstore, and sit down to go through the pages. Allow your mind to wander and wander around with someone else for a few minutes. You'll come back more relaxed and more at ease with your life. If, for any reason, you aren't your style, don't worry. There are plenty of non-fiction titles you could use as well. Find out about our past, or even your own cultural background. Learn languages, construct things, or learn about ways to combat depression. These are all easily accessible to you. You do not have to leave the house as there are a myriad of websites and apps offering discounted or free ebooks that are available for download. There's nothing like the scent of old books I would highly suggest going to the local library. In this way, you'll not only enjoy the bliss of being in a library and books, but be able to show your support to the library.

Music

When you talk about the magic of books and films You are usually given an easy illustration of how to utilize your imagination. Films and books are plots, they feature stories, and they are based on the specific persona. It is possible to imagine yourself as a part of their world, or connect yourself to a character you are familiar with and follow on your journey. Music is completely different. The majority of songs are inspired by a muse or the meaning of their writer or the performer, can be obscure enough to be perceived in different ways by various people. That's why music can have such a profound influence in our daily lives. No matter if you love your music without or with lyrics, you'll find something that resonates with you. One of the greatest things about music is that it has songs for every circumstance you'll ever be in. Every emotion or mood can be expressed through music and these songs can alter your mood and emotions each time you listen to them for a period of time. This is among the reasons that music is commonplace throughout our daily lives.

Chapter 12: Treatment of Depression with Mindfulness Meditation

Mindfulness meditation involves focusing on the sensations and thoughts, without judgement or attachment. When you experience extreme emotions (e.g. in a panic attack or when depression thinking is at its most intense) It is usually because you are caught up in your extreme thoughts about the situation. As you become more involved in your thoughts about the situation, it gets more stressful and you begin to feel like the situation is getting worse, and your feelings get more acute.

The practice of mindfulness can be used to help you shorten the process, untangle yourself from the deformed thoughts and re-connect with reality. This means that you can tackle the issue without psychological pain or emotional reactiveness.

How To Do Mindfulness Meditation

You can practice mindfulness meditation by following these steps:

Pick a location that you like The location you choose must be free from distractions and distractions. It could be near an outside tree or in an area that is quiet in your house. You could also place calming objects or inspiring items such as images of gorgeous locations or flowers on a specialized table. Candles can be added to help soften the light.

Be comfortable If you are going to be stationary for a few minutes at a time. Therefore make sure you are as comfortable as you can. Make sure the temperature in your room is sufficient. You can also purchase pillows, cushions or blankets to help you sit more comfortable, and also to keep warm when your body temperature dips. Wear loose-fitting clothes.

Make a plan for your meditation time Start with 5-10 minutes of quiet and gradually increase the time. In accordance with your abilities to begin, you can start by smaller intervals of time. Setting a timer can be an effective way to make it less likely to keep track of time while you sit. Choose an alarm that has the sound of soft piano or soothing chimes , to serve in the "end of your meditation."

Relax into the meditation posture In addition to the standard posture of the lotus (where you lie with your with your legs crossed) it is also possible to sit in a chair on the floor, lay down, stand or walk. You can experiment various postures until you discover your preferred one. It will feel comfortable to you. If you opt to lay on your back, make sure you do not become sleepy during meditation.

Start to let your mind rest first. It will be more prone to settling and start separating yourself from the events around you. If you've experienced an extremely stressful day, this could be more difficult because you'll begin to think about the things you must do or events that took place. It's normal to be a little unsure Take a few moments and note the emotions when they arise before shifting your attention to the position you are in. Make sure you are comfortable.

Relax for a while Focus on your breath, and take note of your exhalations and inhalations while you breathe. Notice how each breath moves through your body as your lungs expand before releasing the air through your mouth and throat.

Try lengthening and deepening your breath. Deep breathing can assist in relaxing your mind and body. You can still be mindful of your breath throughout the meditation. Watching your breathing can be an effective mindfulness practice.

Be aware that you're not your thoughts. Continue in mind that you are in control over what thoughts and emotions you decide to concentrate on. If you are experiencing unpleasant emotions or thoughts popping out, let them go and refrain from focusing on them. If you notice your mind's stream of thoughts and emotions don't judge yourself. Learn to accept these thoughts and thoughts without judging.

When noises, thoughts or other distractions distract you, try focusing on your breathing: When you concentrate on breathing, balance is the primary focus. You should keep the habit of not judging your thoughts, or even what your meditation experience is like. If you are judging yourself, it can disrupt your meditation practice.

Being distracted or having thoughts about your day are common. The aim is to remain on the present. Your thoughts and emotions can be able to travel back in time or even the future however, your body remains immersed in the present. Therefore, your breathing must always help you stay focused on the present moment.

You can be mindful while working on your normal tasks:

Make sure you eat mindfully so that you are able to slow down and take in the pleasures of your food. Eat an apple in a mindful manner. This will assist you in avoiding eating food to get rid of the stress.

Look at it, observing its texture, shape or any other marks that could be left on the apple.

Try to feel the apple with your hands.

Bring the apple to your face, and then try to smell it. You will observe the way your body reacts. Are you experiencing an increased desire to try it? Are you in a state of excitement?

Take a bite of the apple and make a note of the way it feels, how it taste, or if chewing is enjoyable.

Be mindful when walking It has been instances of people being injured on the roads due to mindlessness caused by depression. One of the best ways to relax and avoid these situations is to walk with a mindful approach.

Walk around and pay focus on how you feel walking as you notice the stretching or bend and muscle movement. The pace you walk at should be slow to allow you to concentrate on your movements and sensations you feel as your feet touch the ground. Try walking in barefoot, so your feet are able to experience more sensations like the temperature of the ground and its surface.

Take your time brushing your teeth Be aware of the bristles on your toothbrush or the motion of your fingers and try to taste the toothpaste. Remember to return to your breath, and then observe your thoughts and feelings , without any judgement.

Use Self-Compassion to Help Treat Depression

Depression can make you hate yourself and feel that you're no worth, nobody loves you and you be nothing. When you practice speaking to yourself with more kindness and lovingly, you will begin to feel more positive about yourself and that will help you overcome depression more effectively.

If you're practicing self-compassion it is crucial to realize that self-compassion relies on goodwill, not positive emotions: Being nice and encouraging to yourself is a great approach to reduce the pain and suffering, but it does not allow you to control the way things go. Don't make use of this technique to suppress or try to fight the pain because otherwise it will make things worse.

Be aware of the pain and embrace yourself with compassion and compassion, recognizing that imperfections are normal. In the end, wrap yourself with love and affection and offer yourself the comfort and strength to endure the pain and provide the most favorable conditions for growth and transformation.

As you begin to work on self-compassion, the pain you feel can dramatically increase in the beginning. But don't fret; it's called backdraft. It means your heart has opened up the gate to your heart, and love is pouring through as the hurts flow out. If you are practicing self-compassion, you will be a slow learning.

Focus on giving your self unconditional love and compassion and show yourself plenty of love. Create a secure environment of self-love and respect because this will allow you to grow into an integrated compassionate, imaginative, and generous person.

How to become more self-compassionate

You can increase your self-confidence by:

Making a self-compassional mantra: The word mantra can be a word that you repeat for remembrance of your current situation and the goals you have set for yourself. It is possible to create a mantra like "This is a time of discomfort. The human condition is prone to pain. Let me show myself the compassion I require to be compassionate towards myself."

Note down any self-deflections that you have: Write down any words you used to make yourself feel bad about yourself and come up with. Consider if you could use the same phrases to a person you know. Imagine what your friend would have to say and record it in addition. Consider the positive things the person you are writing about would have said.

Write yourself a letter: Imagine yourself as a caring friend. Write a letter to someone else. Ask yourself,"What could a kind and compassionate friend say to me today?" Come back after some time and read the letter and then accept it.

Scheduled Activity To Treat Depression

The activity scheduling program helps you participate in a sport or activity that you do normally not take part in. It is a great way to bring rewarding activities back to your daily routine. There is some argument to suggest that feeling inactive is not the sign of depression; instead, it's the reason behind depression. So the less you engage in and the more depressed feel. The more depressed you feel more you don't perform.

How To Manage Scheduling Activities

Activity scheduling can help you accomplish something , even when you don't feel like it. It is possible to schedule your activities according to the following:

Begin to record and monitor your daily activities after a week.

Create a table like the one illustrated on the next page. Input hour-long time slots on the left side, and write each day's name in the top.

Mon Tue Wed Thu Fri Sat Sun

8-9 am

9 - 10 am

10-11 am

You must ensure that you cover the entire day from hour to hour.

Keep track of your most important actions throughout the week for each hour:

Simply write your activities down. This exercise will allow you to create a baseline of your activity which will enable you to keep track of your progress over the coming months.

Rate and identify pleasure and mastery activities: Take a look at the tasks you have written above and follow the steps:

Consider asking yourself "Has the event brought me any enjoyment?" If so write "P" and then rate the pleasure-inducing activity between 1-10 which is where 1 is the minimum and 10 is extreme pleasure.

Similar to mastery-related activities, but use "M" in place of "P." Mastery tasks involve taking charge of yourself or others. You can assess the feeling of achievement you have achieved in each exercise on a scale from 1-10, where 1 represents the lowest and 10 is the most satisfying feeling of accomplishment.

Note: It is important to note that the scale isn't measuring what you have achieved objectively or what you could have accomplished prior to becoming depressed. It simply takes into consideration how difficult the task was when you consider your emotions.

Achieving both pleasure and difficult activities will let you know if your life is off equilibrium. You might notice that a lot of things that you used to love aren't part of your week! The pleasure ratings can provide specific information on the things that can boost your mood as well as those are still enjoyable. Mastery ratings let you know that you're working to do your best even when you're not in a great mood. It's possible that you're not the same level of efficiency as prior to depression however, what you're accomplishing is a real accomplishment.

Plan activities: Now, you can enhance your mastery and enjoy activities that you have on your agenda.

Find 10 hours on your schedule of activities where you're doing an optional task (you don't feel any pleasure or sense of accomplishment).

If you have one or two of these hours each day, plan leisure or mastery activities to fill the profitable hours. Activities for pleasure could include:

Gardening

Going out for a meal

Planning a trip for the weekend or planning for a trip

Music listening

Chat rooms on the Internet

Exercises

Plays/movies

Visits to family or friends

You can record 20 fun activities that you have created on your own. Take the time to think of things that you have liked at the moment. You can also list 20 activities that you've enjoyed in the past that you could enjoy in the future. Many of these may seem boring, but don't worry about it.

Pick 5-7 activities that you enjoy and arrange them for the following week's chart of activities: It is possible to add 1 new mastery exercise each day. The activities that are mastery-focused include:

Cutting hair

Journaling in a journal

Change the oil in your car

Going to work

Resolving a problem

Laundry

Supervising children's nighttime

Helping your child with homework

Bathing

Making hot food

You could also develop your own list of tasks that will bring you a sense your own accomplishment.

Choose 5-7 tasks from the mastery list and incorporate them in your next week Avoid attempting an activity for mastery that could be too difficult. Simply review the hours of the first week's schedule when you're unproductive and depressed. Replace them with mastery-based activities to achieve a sense of accomplishment. Consider your daily activity schedule as an appointment with someone whom you like, admire and do not wish to disappoint them.

The third week of your training is likely to be similar to the second week, with 5-7 fun activities, and 5-7 additional mastery exercises.

In subsequent weeks, you should set an objective to add 7 additional enjoyment and mastery activities to your weekly schedule. You can keep as many of your favorite old activities as you like. You can stop any exercise which did not go well. Keep track of things you've been avoiding as a way to gauge your the activities you can master. For example, if you put off washing dishes, schedule an appointment on your weekly schedule of activities and get it done.

When you are creating your activity schedules Begin to predict the level of satisfaction or accomplishment in the first day each week. You should be able to predict how the activities you're planning will affect your mood.

Create a blank weekly schedule of activities and create your own new activities for mastery and pleasure during the coming week. Utilize the scale 1-10 to assess the level of achievement or satisfaction you'll accomplish and circle the number when you fill in the calendar.

Note your real-life evaluations alongside your predictions in circles throughout the week. You'll notice that real fulfillment and satisfaction feel better than your predictions. It is because depression causes you to feel negative. When you contrast the level of success or joy you attain to your hopes you'll see how depression alters your perspective.

There are times when you find yourself feeling that you don't have the time to complete something new during your day. Keep in mind that your daily schedule of activities can assist you in beating depression. Eliminating or limiting certain of the activities that you usually perform could be the best option to boost your happiness and satisfaction.

Chapter 13: Keep Positive Attitude

Remember the trick to trick your subconscious mind to be positive and happy by having a smile for 10 minutes every day? The reason this works is that your subconscious mind receives information and then reacts to it. It doesn't even think about the content or the source It just takes the information and responds. This is the reason why smiling even when it's for no reason whatsoever can to combat anxiety and depression. It's like magic.

You can go further then this in order in order to "trick" your mind into believing that you are satisfied, happy and content. The easiest way to do this is to have a conversation with yourself. There's a bit of a negative connotation attached to having a conversation with yourself, however it's one of the most effective practices I've discovered for myself and my clients to boost happiness, mood, satisfaction and happiness, as well as mood and outlook.

The method is, as with everything else in the book, easy and straightforward to carry out. All you have to do is set aside five to 10 minutes each day to speak positively to yourself. Relax and say things to yourself that result in happiness. Do it in a way that is easy, and do it when you're driving or when you get up in the early morning.

You can tell yourself what your subconscious mind wants to listen to: I'm content. More than the majority of people do in their lives. It's possible that I don't love my job, but at least I'm not a slave to it. Although I might not be the most wealthy or rich as I would like to be, but I'm working on making a change and at the very least have enough money to live off. I have friends and family who are there for me and love me. It's not the most luxurious or expensive automobile, however I have a vehicle that can get me to where I want to get to. I've had to deal with anxiety and depression at times, however today I'm in charge of my situation and working towards a life I would like which will bring me and keep me satisfied.

It may seem absurd however, I've personally employed positive self-talk in order to double my earnings, improve my relationships, bring more joy and prosperity within my own life and create an ideal future for myself and those I cherish. Positive self-talk has made enormous changes in my clients' perspective regarding life, their mental outlook as well as their happiness and their sense of self-worth and satisfaction.

It is probably to be one of the effective methods you can employ to combat anxiety and depression Don't dismiss this method because it appears ridiculous! The effects will be apparent rapidly. The subconscious mind plays more of a influence on your happiness and daily life, than what your brain and you must ensure that you are filled with the positive thoughts you'd like to keep throughout your life.

Do Something Different

Similar to how routines can be a wonderful option to beat depression, it could also be an obstacle to happiness. Routine is an excellent method of gaining the impression that you're in control of your life. in order, but you need to be able to vary your daily routine. Repeating the same routine repeatedly results in monotony, a feeling of being stuck and eventually higher levels of depression.

The best way to beat the monotony of your life? Find something different! No matter how huge or complicated it may be the most important thing is that you attempt something completely new. You could pick on a new instrument, start learning a new language, or start engaging in a new pastime. There are many options to choose from, ranging from costly to completely free. All you have to do is select something and begin. It could be as frequently as every day, every week, or perhaps every month.

When you try something new, it provides you with the sensation of change. This allows you to recognize that you'll never be the same person that you're in now. Things will change. There will be times when you're not depressed You won't always be stressed. Change is among the best methods to gain the feeling of rejuvination every day.

Have Fun!

One of the main causes for anxiety and depression in America and a majority of most renowned countries around the globe is work and the strain of responsibility to earning money as well as paying for food, clothing, as well as your vehicle in addition to maintaining and maintaining your home, as well as spending generally. There is a huge concentration and attention on the day-to-day grind. Everyone seems to be too caught up in the race and making a living that they neglect to live. Don't allow this to happen to your!

Have a weekend once a month or a single day per week to go out and for a fun time. Engage in something that is completely enjoyable and is solely for joy and happiness. Something that lets you get rid from the pressure to earn money. It could be anything such as mountain biking, take a stroll on the beach, do yoga, take an excursion, take an easy ride in your car, or to a coffee shop with a buddy.

We're so deeply entangled in the pursuit of an income that we often forget about the enjoyment of life. Life isn't about making money and staying alive, it's about enjoying yourself by doing the things you love and that bring you joy. It's true that it's essential to make a profit and sustain your current lifestyle however if you're spending all your time worrying over expenses and bills, then what's the reason?

You should disconnect from your life every now and then to recharge. It is essential to get away from your work and money, as well as all things that bring you back to your daily routine. Get out and have fun. Take advantage of your time, as everyone has a small amount of it around 80 years later and we're done and we don't get more. It is essential that at least some time is spent being relaxed and happy.

It's crucial to recognize that fun and relaxation shouldn't always involve drinking a glass of wine or watching television. Smoking cigarettes, alcohol and food overindulgence are now the main sources of relaxation to lots of people. It's fine to have a few drinks once some time, but you must be a bit adventurous and discover something completely new. Enjoy a day at the beach with your loved one and chat, enjoy lunch, take a relaxing bike ride with your friend or take a stroll in your backyard and read. The new ways to relax are essential. When you're having fun with yourself , that your batteries are recharged and depression is slowly dissolving from your. Enjoy life to the fullest!

Help Someone else

Another method to increase the feeling of importance and satisfaction in your life is to simply give something to others, and not expect any reward from them in exchange. Whatever selfishness one may be the feeling is always good to help the person they love.

As with everything else the task could be as easy as cooking breakfast for one of your family members or helping your friend move into the new place, or removing the snow of the sidewalk of your neighbor after you're done the task on your own. It doesn't need to be a huge act of selflessness...all you have to do is think of something small with someone else.

It is natural to focus on yourself most of the time, since ultimately you're the only one that you are accountable to. Each of us must ensure that we're surviving and prospering, but this self-centeredness could cause you to believe that the world is yours and all you have to be focused on. Giving that attention to another person will not only make their day, it also helps your mind to understand that there's something more than what that you're currently dealing with.

One morning I found myself in bad mood. I'd had no sleep the night prior and I had to get to work but did not want to go do so, and I had not exercised the previous morning. The day was looking grim and I was unable to break out of the depression I was in. I entered the kitchen, where my mother and sister were seated, and for some reason, I performed an unintentional dance when I made my way into. They laughed and I smiled. A small and easy act, such as making someone laugh immediately brought joy to my day. And I had an amazing remainder of the day, too.

Also, it does not matter how big or small your gesture. When you're focused to make someone smile and helping someone it is certain that your day will not be brighter even if it's just a tiny less. Set a goal to do something to help others every day of the week, and continue the practice even after the week has ended. In combination with everything else you read in the book will help reduce your anxiety, decrease your depression and provide you with satisfaction and satisfaction throughout your day. It's that easy!

Be aware that things change

It's easy to concentrate heavily in the moment because...well we live within the moment. There's not much else to focus our attention on as the present and the things we're doing and thinking about takes up most of our attention.

The most important aspect to keep in mind is that things can change such as your anxiety and depression. You might feel depressed this day but that's not to suggest that you'll feel the exact way next week or tomorrow. Depression is a normal thing, but knowing that it is possible, happens and will alter is essential of overcoming depression.

You may think that depression is a stumbling block and overcome, but it isn't. It's not always the case but recollecting this will help to get rid of the feelings.

Sometimes , it can seem as if it's hopelessand you'll never eliminate the sadness, depressed, down-hearted feeling. It's not. It is a fact that depression occurs and then it fades out of sight, and might return for a brief time. One of the most crucial things to keep in mind is that it will eventually disappear, and that there is a conclusion soon. It should make you feel at least a bit at the thought that you may feel anxious or depressed in the present but it will pass and there will be an time in the near future when joy and happiness prevail once more. If you are unable to rid yourself of it then just keep going and trust that it will be over.

Express your gratitude

When you're struggling and depressed, the last thing you're inclined to do is think about all the things you're grateful for, however you have to push yourself to make it happen. Be grateful on a regular routine, either in the mirror during your commute, you're walking or working. All you have to do is consider the things that happen in your life to which you're thankful.

The reason this happens very well is that we take what we are blessed with for granted. It's not often that you encounter someone who is continually grateful for what they have instead of becoming bitter for everything they do not have. This is how we operate naturally, however as with other things, you can modify this.

It's as easy as reciting what you're grateful for. If you're not able to locate something you're truly grateful for, think about the aspects of those things that you're grateful for. As an example, you may not like your job but at least you've got one which is payed, and it gives you food. Most people don't know that they have work.

What this tells your subconscious mind is that it communicates to it what is most important and what to concentrate on. There's a part of the brain known as"reticular activating system (RAS) that regulates awakeness and determines what's essential enough to concentrate on. One good illustration of this is when you purchase the exact make and model vehicle and you suddenly notice them everywhere on the road , even though you weren't before. They've always been there, naturally however, now the particular make and model is important to you, and your RAS determines that it's significant and significant enough that you should focus on the specific make and model of vehicle.

Your RAS determines what you're focused on and when you inform your RAS and your subconscious mind repeatedly and over again what you're grateful for, it goes to search for more reasons to be grateful for. Your mind suddenly becomes positive all by itself and depression and anxiety have absolutely no space in a mind that is positive.

What's more amazing than this new way of thinking is that it helps train and prepares your mind to anticipate positive outcomes in the near future. You will notice that the environment around you is a more positive one than you previously believed. This can make a significant impact on your life, to see the world around you in a positive light.

The only thing you have to do to make a difference is to consider 10 things you're grateful each day. They could be the exact things that you did the previous day or even 10 different things...just consider the 10 things to be thankful for that makes you feel happy or grateful. Record them down if that's what you'd like while recording the daily tasks.

Stay in contact

If depression or anxiety sets in, the natural reaction is to isolate yourself from the world. It's either not a good idea to have others to see us as depressed or others to "have to cope with" the depression. This is not a viable solution in the long run.

It's possible that when you begin to begin to feel anxiety or depression coming in, you're ready to get rid of the company that you're in and separate yourself. It could even aid. But you must be able to avoid isolation for long durations of time.

We are naturally social even if you think or believe you're not social. People are a pleasure to be around as well as social interaction, no matter what they are, can improve our mental state. Just being around others can reduce a sense of despair and more a feeling of belonging. If you're apprehensive about yourself, then you'll feel more lonely and overwhelmed. Therefore, avoid isolation when anxiety or depression are affecting you.

Being alone with people can be enough for a lot of people to experience the feeling of belonging. So you can imagine how helpful it is to communicate with the people you know about how you're feeling. Find someone who is near to you, and speak to them about what you're feeling. It's possible to be resistant initially however, you'll be able to benefit from it even if it's just small.

If you're not comfortable discussing anxiety or depression with those closest to you, think about speaking to an therapist. A simple conversation even if it's about your mood or feelings could drastically alter the state of depression you are in. You might feel that you'd prefer to be in a room by yourself But you can overcome your feelings and embrace the reality that social interactions are among our natural coping strategies.

Chapter 14: To Manage Depression Related to Work

The degree of depression differ. Depression can be serious or mild. It is good to know that both kinds are treatable. Major depression is treatable by taking antidepressants. However, it is important to note that even though many antidepressants have the same effect but not all are able to treat the same adverse effects.

Another approach to treating major depression is to use cognitive therapy for behavioral disorders. This treatment method has the same effect as antidepressants, however using a combination of both methods could be more efficient. Interpersonal therapy is also utilized. It involves revisiting traumas from the past and enhancing emotional awareness.

Minor depression However, minor depression it can be cured by itself. Patients suffering from mild depression should take self-care, or seek help from a professional. Self-management resources that provide instructions on how to deal with issues and deal with depression are accessible through the internet.

If you suffer from minor depression, it is possible to seek professional help and receive therapy that is focused on coaching adaptive strategies for reversing the negative thinking process as well as managing mood, coping with stressors and improving relationships.

Interventions could also be required to stop your mild depression from becoming worse. If you do not find interventions to be effective then you can seek specific treatments, like cognitive behavioral therapy as well as antidepressant medications.

Antidepressant Medicines

There are many antidepressant drugs that are available. The most often prescribed antidepressants are known as Selective Serotonin Reuptake Inhibitors , or SSRIs. They tend to be non-sedative and suitable for the majority of patients.

Serotonin as well as Noradrenalin Reuptake Inhibitors, also known as SNRIs are also used in a variety of. Contrary to antidepressants of the past they have side effects that are less. They are generally given to those suffering from severe depression.

Reversible inhibitors or Monoamine oxidase or RIMAs are not sedative and have less adverse negative effects. They might not be suggested to patients suffering from depression, but they can be helpful for those suffering from sleep disorders and anxiety.

TriCyclic Antidepressants, or TCAs are also effective however, their negative side negative effects can be dangerous. They can also reduce blood pressure.

Monoamine Oxidase Inhibitors , also known as MAOIs could have undesirable consequences. This is why they should be used only in specific cases.

You can also try Noradrenaline-Serotonin Specific Antidepressants or NaSSAs. They're relatively new and can assist you to get better sleep and reduce anxiety levels. But, they can be a cause of weight gain.

Noradrenalin Reuptake Inhibitors (NARIs) NARIs are made to selectively react to noradrenalin, which is an important chemical found within the brain. In contrast to other antidepressants, they aren't very likely to induce sleepiness. They can, however, cause sleepiness, increase the sweating and cause the process of urinating more difficult following the first doses.

Simple Work Depression Busters

Like we said earlier self-help therapy can be used for mild depression. If you're looking to feel better, consider these simple but efficient methods to get rid of depression at work. It's possible to make a difference. prove worthwhile at the end of the day.

If you're struggling at work, it is likely that you consider quitting your job every day. You shouldn't do it. In the event that you try, you'll be feeling worse. What causes this? If you decide to quit your job, you'll have more time and this can lead to contemplate how you feel about your work.

Additionally the depression could get worse as you pay your next water, electric or phone invoice. Since you're no longer employed or have an employment, you don't have a steady income. This means your phone as well as your water and electricity may be cut off and you may be evicted from your home at any time if you don't pay. Furthermore, you'll feel more lonely and sad since you'll have no person to communicate with. Everyone else is working at the moment, at the end of the day.

In addition, it is important to be aware of techniques for relaxation. Meditation, yoga as well as visual visualization are some of the most popular relaxation methods used by people to relax themselves. In the break you could take a break in a peaceful tranquil spot at work and be in a quiet space with your thoughts. Breathe deeply and exhale. You can also enjoy soothing music to ease your tension.

If you're looking to relax then you might want to get away from your phone. Because of modern technology, it's easy to connect with others through mobile phones. But, these devices can be a source of anxiety and depression. The constant stream of messages may be exhausting.

Also, getting calls from different people could make you feel stressed. Therefore, instead of reading and responding to messages constantly You should take a break. Switch off your mobile for a bit and attempt to be relaxed. You'll be amazed at how peaceful you feel without these devices.

Being unorganized and messy is a great way to stress yourself out. It is therefore important to organize your schedule and adhere to it. Use a planner or organizer where you make notes, important notes, reminders, and other tasks. This is particularly helpful when you have a busy schedule. Making sure that your work is completed according to the priority levels can help you stay organised and efficient.

Also, you should tidy your workspace to ensure your work environment is in good order. Being in a messy office could make you feel sad. You won't be able to locate what you require easily, and you may be exhausted just gazing at the cluttered pile of papers and other items that are piled up on the desk. You could also beautify your workplace by putting a potted plant in it or photos that you have framed. In addition, you could have lighting that makes your workplace more bright.

Signs and symptoms for "Burnout" and How you can do to prevent the occurrence.

To prevent depression that is severe You must be able recognize signs of burnout. Robert Wicks, a psychologist who studies burnout, states that signs of burnout at work include anger and helplessness, apathy and impatience, as well as a decrease in confidence in yourself and your self, depression and a lack of joy.

You could say you suffer from a level 1 burnout when you are experiencing moderate signs of depression. The level of your burnout has increased as your symptoms worsen and get more intense. If your burnout rate increases further and your symptoms become more severe, they will become chronic. Then you start developing physical illnesses. To prevent any further injury, it is recommended to take a break from your job.

Have a getaway and visit new places. After all day you should have time off. The time away from the daily grind will help you relax and help you become more productive. The time off can help prevent burnout. When you get back to work, you'll be able to perform your obligations more effectively.

You must also begin to have an active social life If you've been focused on your work all the years. Every week, you may go to the club or hang in a bar along with your colleagues or friends. Socializing lets you let go of the stress at your job and also allows you to connect with new people.

It is also important to be able to have a social life in addition to your job. You could join the book club, participate in a cooking class or even take up activities. It is not necessary to be confined to working at the office. There's more to life that just work. Making a difference outside of your job can help you become more complete and rounded.

Chapter 15: Anxiety Therapy

These are the methods that are the most popular and highly effective in treating depression and anxiety. Although you might not suffer from a disorder, these therapies can still be helpful in reducing depression and anxiety.

Cognitive-Behavioral Therapy (CBT)

A proven, highly effective treatment that lasts is known as cognitive-behavioral treatment, or CBT. It is focused on identifying, understanding, and changing thought and behaviour patterns. The benefits are typically seen after 12 to 16 weeks according to the individual.

In this form of therapy the patient is engaged in their self-care, feels an awareness of his or her own control and gains skills that will be valuable throughout the course of their lives. CBT usually involves discussing the problem and keeping track of appointments, and also completing homework assignments during which treatments are practiced.

Patients are taught skills in therapy sessions but they have to practice the skills often to see improvements.

Therapy for Exposure

A type of CBT that is called exposure therapy, it's an approach for reducing anxiety and fear-related reactions. Therapy is where a patient is slowly exposed to a fearful subject or object, and learns to be less sensitive over time. This kind of therapy has proven to be particularly effective in treating the disorder of obsessive-compulsive and phobias.

Acceptance Therapy and Commitment Therapy (ACT)

Also called ACT, this kind of therapy employs techniques of accepting and mindful (living in the present and being present in the moment without judgment) as well as determination and change in behavior as a means to deal with negative thoughts emotions, feelings, and feelings. ACT gives you the ability to be able to accept the experiences, place them in a new context and gain greater clarity on your personal values, and then make a commitment to the necessary behavior change.

Dialectical Behavioral Therapy (DBT)

It is a method of combining cognitive-behavioral practices and concepts drawn from Eastern mediation, such as dialectical behavior therapy, also known as DBT which combines acceptance with transformation. DBT involves group and individual therapy to develop mindfulness and also skills for interpersonal efficiency, managing anxiety, and managing emotions.

Interpersonal Therapy (IPT)

It is commonly called IPT interpersonal therapy that is a short-term and supportive psychotherapy that addresses issues with interpersonal relationships with depression among adolescents, adults as well as older adults. IPT generally comprises 12-to-16 one-hour weekly sessions. The first sessions are dedicated to gathering information on the character of a individual's depression and their interactions.

Eye Movement Desensitization and Reprocessing (EMDR)

When certain conditions are met, eye movements can reduce the intensity of thoughts that are disturbing. A procedure called eye movement desensitization and processing or EMDR appears to exert a direct influence on the way the brain process information. It basically helps people see material that is disturbing in a way that is less stressful.

EMDR seems to be like what happens naturally during dreams and the REM (rapid eye movements) sleep. The results of scientific research have established EMDR as an effective treatment in treating posttraumatic stress disorders. Additionally, clinicians have been successful with it in treating anxiety attacks and phobias.

Quoted and not quoted from http://www.adaa.org/

Who is most likely to be Depressed?

The study identified that the following groups were more likely to be able to meet the requirements of major depressive disorder:

Age group 45-64

Women

Blacks Hispanics, blacks, non-Hispanic individuals of different races, or multiple races

Individuals who have less than the level of high school education

The couples who were have been married before

Unemployed or find work

People who do not have health insurance coverage

Similar patterns were also observed in those suffering from "other depression" with two differences: adults between the ages of 18-24 were the most likely to experience "other depression" and so are Hispanics (instead of non-Hispanics). CDC

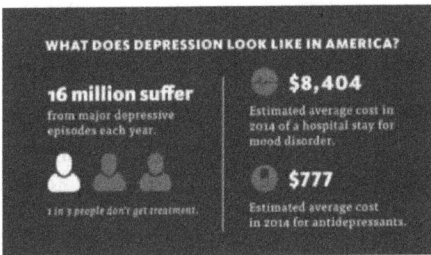

WHAT DOES DEPRESSION LOOK LIKE IN AMERICA?

16 million suffer from major depressive episodes each year.

1 in 3 people don't get treatment.

$8,404 Estimated average cost in 2014 of a hospital stay for mood disorder.

$777 Estimated average cost in 2014 for antidepressants.

This report was revised on March 31, 2011. Since since then, the figures have changed because the foreclosure, housing and economy rates have changed. Today, more persons than there were before struggling from depression and anxiety as jobs become less plentiful and more lose their houses. Children are also suffering from anxiety-related disorders.

When the study was created, there was one out of 10 people was suffering from depression and anxiety. In a study carried out within the United Kingdom, the report is now one of 3 people are suffering from anxiety.Depression Alliance

A lot of people be afflicted by anxiety-related symptoms because they are unable to afford to see a doctor for treatment. There are numerous places which can assist with finances and also a clinics are free and you can attend for more information about the different treatments available.

I found this Infographic on Nerd Wallet at dot com that provides the most recent figures regarding health care for anxiety-related depression for 2013, as well as how the health program will assist financially.

THE DEPRESSION EPIDEMIC
Can Obamacare Fix it?

Depression is a major cost to American society.
The economic burden of depression – in terms of medical
care, missed days of work, chronic health problems, and
deaths – is estimated to have cost $112 billion in 2013.
The Affordable Care Act, or Obamacare, mandates mental
health coverage for millions of Americans.

Therefore, you can expect an opportunity to receive financial assistance in the near future. But, for now you should do more exercise to boost the amount of serotonin in your body. Serotonin is the hormone that assists in mood. When your mood is improved it is possible to be able to see that the end of the rainbow.

Also you'll be able find ways to help yourself even if you're unable to afford medical treatment.

You can also utilize natural remedies and alternative therapies to aid yourself as well as your children.The next chapter will guide you through a variety of ways to combat anxiety and depression.

Chapter 16: Ways To Avoid

Depression Relapse

If you've been through an episode of depression and been treated for it, the first thing you'll want to witness is the possibility of a rebound. Depression is a sour and unappealing that you shouldn't want to share with your most hated adversaries. However, many people suffering from depression do experience relapses in recovery and, in particular, when appropriate measures are not taken to prevent this issue. Here are some steps you can follow to lead an active and healthy lifestyle and prevent a return.

Beware of overloading your brain.

The world has turned into an extremely busy place and many believe that they'll fail if they don't participate in lots of activities. While it's essential to keep engaged, cramming your schedule with too much can cause depression recrudescence. An emotional adversity could cause stress and increases the likelihood of a relapse in depression. It is essential to be aware of your limits and maintain an equilibrium in dealing with issues of daily life. This will help ensure your safety. Take a moment to think about the simplicity of life for your grandparents or your ancestors and how they managed well and their lives were equally important and valuable. Try to emulate the way they lived.

Exercise regularly

Exercise is an integral part of the natural treatment for depression. It can also be beneficial in preventing depression rebound. Regular exercise is an antidepressant and reduces depression associated symptoms. Research suggests that exercise which are combined with meditation could assist in preventing cases of depression and the relapse of depression.

Develop healthy thinking abilities and maintain a positive mindset

The ability to look at life with a positive perspective and cultivating a positive outlook can help you overcome depression triggers. Therapies like cognitive Behavioral Therapy are geared to assist patients suffering from depression in developing an optimistic outlook on himself or herself, as well as life generally. Even though these treatments do not do the job in isolation, patients are able to apply the lessons learned to build a positive perspective regarding issues, and thus overcome actual and imaginary triggers which could cause depression. Whatever may have caused depression or brought it on the ability to develop a positive mindset can serve as a defense against any rebound. Do not draw too much conclusions from the internet and, further try not to judge yourself or a situation with harshness just because you've noticed an aspect that is negative.

Eat proper diet

Food choices can help you keep your mental and physical well-being. For instance, food items that are high in omega-3, with low fat content and high in folic acid can aid in the creation of a positive mood. Other items that can aid in relieving stress include green teas, herbal and black as well as fruits and vegetables. Also, stay away from drinking alcohol, and limit the intake of caffeine-containing food items as part of a healthy diet program.

Get involved in your social circle

A lot of people who suffer from depression tend to live an isolated or lonely life before and throughout their illness. But, establishing trusting and healthy connections can not only in helping recover but also to prevent instances of depression Relapse. Don't be isolated in your own life Instead, make connections to others and appreciate their support and love.

Stop self-blaming

Self-pity and other instances of being overly concerned of the smallest issues within your life can cause depression symptoms. If you're going through the midst of a down time or have a lot to handle It is important to not blame yourself for the problems that happens in your life.

Relax and get a good night's sleep

A good amount of rest and sleep is vital to recovery and avoidance of depression Relapses. Sleeping can help you stabilize your mood as well as reviving your physical and mental health. Sleep deprivation is more likely to fall into depression than people who are able to sleep at night. Sleep is vital to your health, and it is important to never consider it to be a waste of time. A lot of people believe that staying up all night is an indication of lazyness. This is not the case and is one of the most common myths in our busy world. Resting and sleeping properly can allow your body and mind perform at a high level.

It is equally important to make time to engage in activities that bring you joy.

Most often, those suffering from depression tend to cut back on those activities. This could hinder the recovery process. To lead a healthy lifestyle and avoid relapses, you need to make the list of activities that bring you joy about your life. You should engage with them when you see certain warning signs or feel overwhelmed. It doesn't matter if it's swimming or conversing with an acquaintance, or traveling, or participating in a particular activity, make sure you take your time and get the most of those occasions. Remember, overcoming depression is an ongoing process. It is unlikely that you would wish to go back to the dungeon So, stay healthy and feel content.

Chapter 17: Interprting the Groups of Depression Cycle Analysis

1. Superlative Cluster - Score line 0-30.

This is the first instance of depression in which the prospective patient of the depression has been unflinching and unaffected by the nudge of depression. Depression is usually viewed as not attractive and unwelcome at this stage. The waves of depression are reverberating through minds and thoughts, but they are not attract the attention of the mind. In this moment the person is able to offer depression an unmistakable appeal...saying "I know your tricks and I understand your aversions, but there's no way to go here" The person most often is keeping the course of his personality , with an air of calmness without debate. This is the range of vulnerability between 0 and 30. The score is the cluster that defines the individual. Therefore, depression stays from you.

Beware; Do not entertain negative thoughts for even a second. You should immediately ignore. Be aware that negative thoughts are created in the darkroom, and you must reject any thoughts that are contrary to your beliefs.

2. Receptive Cluster score -31-40% line.

The second part of outcomes for depression management. The patient is open, accessible , and accessible. Through subtle methods the mind begins to relax to contemplate certain options, and displaying some curiosity about depressive symptoms. Depression is

Friendly at friendly at Receptive cluster. The fruit of depression is displayed here in the form negative thoughts, thoughts, and fantasies that connect with the real world to create the case. Any person who scores at least 31% is likely to be susceptible to depression. It is possible to begin to confine yourself small increments towards sympathetic thoughts and explanations of your condition. This is what the extension cluster's way of telling you to "extend your tentacles of determination with conviction and a strong faith and allow your influence to make gaps of acceptance both within as well as without" This is a potentially dangerous gap. When you give depression an opportunity to grow, and it could be a serious threat to the integrity of one's own character.

Caution

Do not give up on depression. Don't accept the reason for your depression and stay clear of any evidences or triggers that may be a part of your system. Be careful not to explain things as you think of a plot to make you feel depressed. Shut all the doors to depression- the eye, ear hands, feet, and hand. Your emotions should be preserved and protected from every attack and negative array of thoughts.

3. Indicative Cluster 41-50 Score line for .

The third group of Depression management results. While eating in pieces, the sounds, sights and symptoms of depression are appreciated and accepted. Motives and fantasies are beginning to take root and become a part of the fabric.

The symptoms show up, and depression's symptoms begin to manifest and the course of. Depression starts to dig into the depths of the person and attempting to discover the roots. In the beginning, symptoms begin to appear to oppress the victim. There are internal analyses which can lead to emotional paralysis. Depression symptoms begin to look for perfect cooperation through suggestions that are dominant. The characteristics of specific symptoms become obvious. Depression starts to court agreement with both external and internal stimuli to cause the individual to act in a negative way. The indicator cluster indicates depression's presence as well as the scoring line ranges from 41 percent to 50 percent. It is also known as the Manifestation cluster for depression management.

Caution

Be aware that you've stepped on the wrong foot and the situation could escalate that is way out of the scope of. Get rid of the negative seed that is starting to distract you and snagging your energy away. Get therapy to be certain you're following the proper path, and in the right time. Contact an expert today. Don't make assumptions or wish things go away. It will manifest later.

4.Assertive Cluster-51-60% score line.

It is also the 4th and final cluster of depression management

consequences that lead to the negative self-confidence over the wrong causes. The depression-related mode that erupts from within, causing mental ill-health and creates a haze in the face of a widespread situations. The main focus is the "buying into" of depression within, with regular outbursts at the smallest of triggers external to. The mind becomes saturated, and the victim is adamant looking for the negative motives to debunk a particular circumstance or fact. The evidence is persistance that is noticeable. Depression in this large group does not require an introduction. The multiplication of symptoms in a short time from top to bottom. The person involved is able to provide reasons in the face of obvious circumstances that will further undermine his personal beliefs and goals. The score line is 51-60% which is a remarkable showing the signs of depression. It is impossible to deny the diverse events that take place in your life when you are in a comprehensive cluster.

Caution

However high the degree of vulnerability, you should not be a victim of a falsehood. Be certain that an unnatural person has taken on certain aspects of your life and has taken an unfair advantage on you. Don't be a fool in your own eyes, and never violate internal arguments and ignore the evidence that is in play. Find a Behavioral Therapist who can identify the root of the issue, its implication and damaged that have been caused by the

Antecedent. Be prepared to give up the flimsiest excuses. Don't run on your own in this group, and please be vocal and get out!

The Aggressive Cluster- Score line of 61-70.

The fifth group of results from depression management is marked by more severe confrontation with the victim. Personal assaults are the biggest concern on the list. The victim is liable for the numerous instances of depression, which never seem to diminish. There is hostility inside and out of. The desire to self-destruct and humiliation grows until astonishing failure stares you at us. The internal breakdown can lead to massive addictions that cannot long be controlled and can result in grave damage; this is the norm in this case. The mind is constantly frenzied and emotions are sliced into many different variables-crucial and insignificant. The person is constantly at war with their previous standards and will soon give up on any other poor decisions. People who suffer from depression with aggressiveness tend to fight over everything. They display aggression with no any shame, whether it is in the public or private in the name of asserting their rights. The person who is aggressive has a negative attitude to genuine and good intentions and may be filled with arguments and agitation to take advantage of every opportunity. It is clear the meaning of depression for the person who is at risk and in need of immediate attention. The score range here is between 61 and 70 percent. This is known as the Attention cluster of depression.

Caution

The most honest recommendation here is to seek out the Behavioral Therapist to ensure an entire breakdown of this emotional environment to help rebuild your personality recovery, and ultimately restoration. Because the patient is often unpredictable, it is vital to ensure that the person is constantly monitored and encouraged by a professional. If he is left alone, it could be the final straw even when the victim appears content, his mood could abruptly change after realization of status and frequent conscious.

The Provocative Score Line: Cluster-71-100.

It is the most severe stage of depression, the six stages referred to by the name of "game changer" The emotional trauma of depression is apparent to many since it is now a major problem that is causing conflict with others. Infractions are the norm of the day for this group. While enjoying a certain activities, the person has lost the core of their personality to the point of exhaustion. The person is totally different and is a far cry from the persona at the start. This group is characterized by doubt as well as fear...always in one hazard or another. He presses against his brick walls in all of his private ventures, and enjoys covering his tracks. The insulting gestures always come in the spotlight. The accumulation of aggression from a clusters of words can cause an unnecessary flame that could not only cause the victim to be burned but also

People that surround him. This person is plagued by negative feelings and a sense of impossibility. Because of his temper, the person's speech is often accompanied by inflammatory remarks which could be extremely offending to others.

Caution

This person in this group is seen as a catastrophe waiting to happen. The person in this cluster must be assisted in locating immediate intervention and rehabilitation. Complete withdrawal as an intervention plan for recovery is the most suitable for this individual. The many violations should be identified, tracked and then trimmed away for eventual return to the persona. This will require a series of psychosocial support and more intense monitoring. An ongoing sadness that isn't sustainable can cause the option of suicide If not properly managed.

SummaryofTreatmentMechanisminDepres sion Management

I.Structural Deviation

II. Trend Analysis

III. Root Cause Analysis

IV.Point Analyze Blank.

Chapter 18: Mindfulness and Cbt

One term you might have been hearing about in connection with CBT can be "Mindfulness." But, what exactly is it? Created for those suffering with frequent, repeated and sometimes severe depressions Mindfulness is a combination of CBT techniques using breathing exercises and meditation, visualization, and other similar techniques that allow one to get past stress and into more productive thinking patterns.

Fundamental Concepts

Mindfulness is the ability to not dwell on the past and worry over the coming days. If you're feeling anxious and stressed, you realize that you cannot put it aside. In the case of Mindfulness The goal is to ease your anxiety that is present in the moment by grounding yourself in this moment.

Mindfulness methods are a way to get your mind off of the worry about past events you are no longer able to manage. When you think of an embarrassing incident that occurred or perhaps something that you're concerned will resurface in your mind, it could make it difficult to enjoy the present.

If you're always worried over the unforeseeable future you'll begin to become lost to the present and other people may be aware that you aren't completely present. The thought of the future does not always bring negative thoughts. It's possible to imagine the life you've always thought was impossible or one with extravagant houses or money, as well as friends and family members to offer peace. While these thoughts do not necessarily create anxiety, they could result in depression when you are trying to avoid the present problems by imagining an imagined future that will not come.

Mindfulness refers to any activity that's going draw you away out of these current moments and lead you back to the present, the moment that is the most important. These types of fantasies as well as the patterns of rumination are examples of dissociation.

The effects of dissociation can be crippling. It is possible to be locked in bed that cannot move. In other instances, it may impact your memory.

How Mindfulness can be linked to CBT

Because CBT is all about rewiring your thinking process, Mindfulness will help give you the chance to end unrealistic fantasies before they start. Instead of surrendering to the thoughts of your mind that is not true, a mindfulness technique can aid in bringing you back to reality.

At times, people begin to separate from the situation because they don't want face a particular problem. If you're feeling affected by someone or something and you are unable to think about it, you may mentally separate your self from the situation and imagine another thing. This change in perspective may be helpful for a short time however you're not addressing the root of your issue. It is important to learn how to utilize CBT techniques for mindfulness to help you prepare for this disassociation attempt.

How Mindfulness Training Can Help

Did you ever sit through an entire class and thought "I have to be attentive. I must pay attention." And then you realize that an hour has passed the class is over and you realise that you were imagining what you'd do during the weekend, or maybe you thought of an excursion to the tropical region. While you were not paying attention in class your mental state was different. place and when you try to focus, it's more difficult than it would be if you been paying attention.

Mindfulness can help bring you back into the classroom. Sometimes we're aware of what is to be attentive however, we may not necessarily notice it when we begin to daydream. We don't always realize the fact that you're dissociating until later when you are able to ask yourself where you are, or what's happened in the last few minutes. If we are dissociating too frequently negative effects can be observed, including anxiety as well as confusion and loss of memory.

Mindfulness

It is similar to meditation however it doesn't need to be done in the same manner. It is possible to be mindful even when you are at the cash machine at work. It is possible to practice mindfulness when you are engaged in an exchange with a friend. It's also possible to practice mindfulness even when you're lying on your couch at your home. There are many ways for people to be mindful and there aren't specific rules for when and when you should do mindfulness. It's entirely dependent on the situation and you where you're trying to become aware.

There are many ways of being aware and, as you learn more, you'll be able to develop a strategy that you have developed your own. There is no guarantee that every person will be able to determine which of these strategies is effective for their particular situation, so make sure you pick the one that's most suitable for you. These strategies can be employed at any time you're sitting on the couch, stressing about something out that of your reach. If you're trying to sleep but your thoughts of depression won't quit take a moment to be aware.

Additionally, if you're attending a celebration and are concerned about how you appear or what you're saying to other people Be aware. If you observe something that makes you feel uncomfortable however you can't get out of the scene, try to be aware. If you ever find yourself feeling like you require more than what's readily available it's a good idea to try practicing Mindfulness. It might seem intimidating and intimidating, but it's your responsibility to try the best you can to stay grounded and not be entangled in your intrusive and intrusive, deformed thoughts and negative ones.

Be aware when doing these exercises, the moment your mind begins to wander back to thoughts of anxiety do not punish yourself. Do your best to redirect your thoughts towards the present moment. It can be difficult initially.

The more you apply these strategies the easier it will become to remain focused on the present moment and not drift to the future or get trapped in your past. You'll develop a greater awareness of the need to continue focussed on the "now" and not think about any other thing that causes anxiety.

Group Mindfulness is crucial also. If you work in a corporate space with lots of individuals, then you are aware that sometimes you take on the stress of others, causing your own stress to rise. If Mindfulness practices are utilized within a group, it can aid in the overall health of everyone.

Games can be a great way to keep your mind in check. Explore free games on your phone you can try that can assist you in reducing anxiety. If you're feeling stressed it is possible to engage in the game, rather than contemplating your worries. In a setting with a crowd or even in a personal sense puzzles are great methods to keep you focused. It is possible to put one on a table during an event to distract people when activities don't seem as lively.

Find ways you can incorporate games into your everyday activities. Instead of watching television after dinner, engage in games with your loved ones to distract everyone from the depressing thoughts. You can also try sudoku, word searches, and crosswords for something to make use of your hands. Coloring books for adults are excellent also.

Relaxed Detective

This is a great practice to help you center yourself and get you into an enlightened state. Imagine your self as a detective searching for clues. Take note of the details of the surroundings. Take note of the colors of the surrounding area, the sky and the grass or the art and photographs if you happen be inside. Be aware of the people in the area. Do they look tall? Short? Take note of hair color and style. Inquiring into the details in your life as if you were a detective could help you get you back on track.

Quote Mantra

Keep a list of your most-loved quotes to recite in your mind when you're stressed or need to achieve an efficient, healthy mindset. In the Tao I-Ching has some good ones, for example.

"Sixteen spokes join on the wheel's hub however, it's not the spokes, however. They are what make the wheel effective. It is rather the empty space in the middle. The artist can design a beautiful vase, however, it's not the vase that is crucial, but rather the empty space within it that you'll fill."

Quotes such as this can help you focus and remain focused.

Fake Yawn

Have you ever seen someone close to you yawn and then you realize that you are crying too? It's happened to everyone and it is quite beneficial for getting an instant and powerful dose of mindfulness. Do an unintentional, slow smile and you will cause this to happen in your mind. It gives you a quick sensation of a peaceful or relaxed state. this small amount is often the only thing you require to maintain your concentration.

Body Scan

The technique is typically performed by a professional, however it can be performed by yourself also. It is recommended to lay on your back with your holding your palms to your sides. The process begins by focusing the breath. Pay attention to how you breathing before focusing on the sensation on your feet, and then your legs, then up down your body.

Be aware of the sensation of moving your toes, and also the feeling of the mat under your feet. Notify any pains or aches while you examine your body. After you've scanned your body this way and come to your head, close by observing the way your scalp feels against the pillows. When you open your eyes, you'll feel relaxed and rejuvenated.

Mindfully Seeing Mindfully

This practice is designed to help you reach an awareness state as well as enhancing your imagination. It is quite relaxing and beautiful after you have completed the technique. Find a place that is comfortable. It could be in your home while gazing at the outside or in a quiet spot in nature that is close to your home. It must be a private area to ensure that you don't get interrupted and can enjoy the exercise to the fullest. The following part is straightforward in its explanation, however you'll find that how to do it requires some time.

See the world around you and be absorbed by the particulars. Contrary to

"Relaxed detective," it is not going to measure the details in a way that empowers instead, you're likely to be able to appreciate their beauty. If you are looking at the dog and you are not considering "dog," focus on the manner in which it walks and the colour that its fur. The trees and flowers turn browns, greens, yellows, as well as all the other colors you can see all over the spectrum. They transform into the motion winds impart to them.

When we take away the names we have for things and focusing our attention on their actual essence it is possible to achieve an enlightened state of mind. This is similar to making up our own names for the things we see every day and placing them in a diffuser similar to the light that is reflected in a prism, in order to observe the range of the things they comprise to appreciate their beauty in a new way. Although this may seem obscure, it actually has a extremely practical benefits from a logic perspective. It helps you relax and teaches your brain to quickly evaluate the various components of a thing , so you are able to appreciate and recognize the thing it. "That's not a flower; it's an orange circle that is made up by tiny, orange-colored dots that have smalldark contrasts the bright yellow ovals, seated on the emerald-colored high stilts." Take a look at this. The art of breaking down a thing into its constituents can not only provide you with the ability to meditate instantly that you can control, but it will also allow you to dissect the most complex thoughts you have by virtue of having been practicing this method. It's a good one to keep.

Becoming Mindful

This type of exercise is typically performed in a group, however, with couples who are extremely open and close to each other (or want to be) this is an extremely beneficial technique to attain a meditative state of awareness and understanding as well as with one another. The process begins by sitting to one another. Every person talks, without interruption in a single sentence, about something they are anxious about and also something they are eager to enjoy. After the first person has finished and the next person finishes, they talk about their individual stress as well as the thing they're looking for pleasure from.

The person who is speaking at the moment should concentrate on how they feel when speaking and what they're saying, such as how their brain is racing as well as how their body is feeling. They should also be focused on the position of the other person when they speak. The listener should pay attention to how they feel when listening and also on the body language. Therefore, body language can be learned. This is sufficient to be useful throughout the exercise however there's more to gain by this technique.

At the end of the session, each participant recalls the experience it was for them to speak and listen. Consider these points What did I feel during my conversation? While listening? Was my mind wandering in any way? Do I ever feel like judged or give judgement?

For couples, a great ending could be for both to repeat what the other stated in your own language. There should not be any judgments made however, some affirmation is possible to give. Some examples of closing remarks include: "Yes, that is exactly what I wanted to convey" or "I am not sure that I understood the whole story, but we'll keep trying to improve our communication to ensure that we all get heard."

Do not expect instant results However, with this method mindfulness and closeness can be increased within the structure of the couple. As with all worthwhile things there is a bit of work involved, but you'll enjoy the outcomes.

Life Savers

Start by taking the first candy roll apart and assign a specific moment of happiness or success to each color of your candy pile.

Try each flavor before you choose it, as it is crucial to get the desired result.

If you're feeling confused and overwhelmed Take an empty Life Saver out of your bag and note the color and then try it. Imagine the joyous moment you've connected to it. Do not think about it too much, simply take a bite and imagine your ideal location, time or moment. Savour it, relish the sweet treat and don't dwell on the issue as long as your Life Saver is over.

The ability to take a moment to focus on positive things to do can help return to a rational and positive attitude to life. Making a mental note within the candy will aid in reliving this memory instantly with a tangible object. Additionally the candy can be taken anywhere.

Five senses

"Five senses" is another fantastic method that is based on nothing more than your body. To use this technique make sure you don't stand up and reach for objects instead, simply visualize them in your mind. This technique will guide you through all five senses, which includes the ability to see, hear, feel, smell, and taste. Also, you will be counting on the fiveth day, so you will have less chance for you of being interrupted by distracting thoughts.

Begin by identifying five items you observe. They could be anything from five to five and you have to choose them with your eyes and your brain. Perhaps it's the sofa right in front of you or the table carrying all your belongings.

Next, you should find four objects that you could touch. Perhaps it's your own leg, or maybe the blanket that wraps around your body. Then, you can pick out three things you can hear. Perhaps the wind is banging at the windows or perhaps you hear a barking dog out the window.

Look for two things you are able to smell. It is possible that you are unable to smell anything at all, for example, perfume or candles however, maybe the sofa the one you're on smells or maybe you live in the vicinity of a coffee shop.

Then, choose something you are able to smell. You should not actually taste this item, but there's something in the environment that you are in which is a taste What is it? What are you capable of identifying this item? Repeat this exercise as many times as it is necessary to stay focused on the present.

Conclusion

Depression is a ailment and it can affect your daily routine change the way you conduct yourself and interact with others, and suppressing joy or the positive feelings you be feeling. It is possible that you feel depressed and unable to cope or prefer to give up, but I would like to remind you that you're not the only one. Many millions of all walks of life regardless of age, gender and race who suffer from this debilitating disease that doesn't just affect you , but also the community around you. If you were determined enough to take the step to actually overcome the dark feelings and thoughts that you might have, there will be a multitude of people willing to be there to support you and fight together. Apart from the calming help of your family and acquaintances There are a variety of organizations that can help you. Depression is reversible. There are treatments you can pick from that can effectively lift you out of the darkness that you're in.

I am very proud of you. The fact that you have downloaded this book is an important step for you or someone you love who might be depressed clinically. Being aware of the subject is an additional weapon to fight depression.

Don't forget that your lives are a gift and you must safeguard it. There are many reasons to keep going on your path. Don't be ashamed or shy about seeking help and this isn't just for selfishness, but rather because you are entitled to get your life.